DETOX!

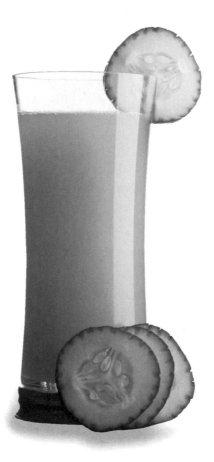

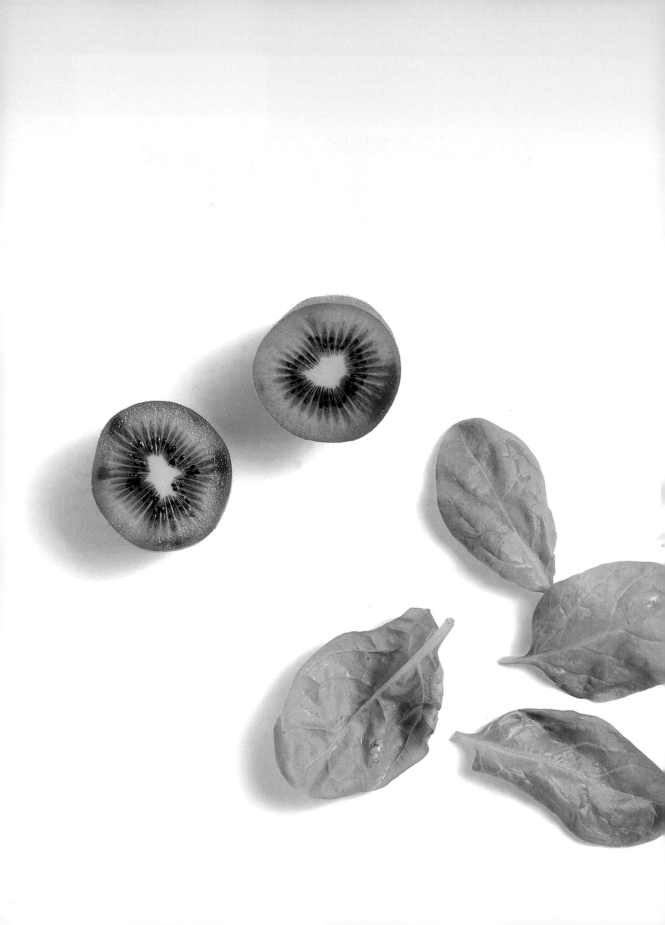

DETOX!

How to Cleanse and Revitalize Your Body, Your Home and Your Life

By the editors of Rodale Health Books

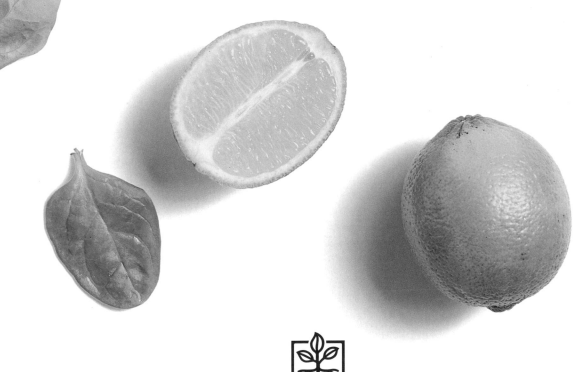

RODALE

This edition first published in the UK in 2006 by
Rodale International Ltd
7–10 Chandos Street
London W1G 9AD
www.rodalebooks.co.uk

Printed and bound in the UK by CPI Bath using acid-free paper from sustainable sources.

1 3 5 7 9 8 6 4 2

A CIP record for this book is available from the British Library

ISBN 13: 978-1-4050-9336-1
ISBN 10: 1-4050-9336-6

This edition distributed to the book trade by Pan Macmillan Ltd

This book was created from material first published in *The Purification Plan*, published in the USA by
Rodale Inc. Rodale International wishes to acknowledge with thanks the many experts who contributed to
The Purification Plan and regret that space in this abridged edition did not allow inclusion of all their names.

The recipes Barley with ginger and broccoli and Fenugreek kichari on page 107 are courtesy of the
Himalayan International Institute of Yoga Science and Philosophy of the USA.

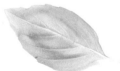

Notice

This book is intended as a reference volume only, not as a medical manual. The information given here is
designed to help you to make informed decisions about your health. It is not intended as a substitute for any
treatment that may have been prescribed by your doctor. If you suspect that you have a medical problem,
we urge you to seek competent medical help. Mention of specific companies, organizations, or authorities in
this book does not imply endorsement by the publisher, nor does mention of specific companies,
organizations, or authorities imply that they endorse this book.

Internet addresses and telephone numbers given in this book were accurate at the time it went to press.

Detox! was created for Rodale International by
Amazon Publishing Ltd.
Editors: Jill Steed, Maggie Pannell, Anna Brandenburger
Designers: Vivienne Brar, Stuart Perry, Maggie Aldred
Nutritionist: Jane Griffin
Consultants: Dr Sheena Meredith, Dr Ann Walker
Photography of recipes pages 102–130: photographer Hugh Johnson,
   home economist Bridget Sargeson, art director Luis Peral

For Rodale International
Managing Editor: Miranda Smith
Design Manager: Jo Connor
Production: Sara Granger
Repro: Acumen Colour Ltd., London
Photographs of exercises: Mitch Mandel

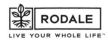

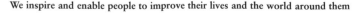

We inspire and enable people to improve their lives and the world around them

Contents

Detoxification in a healthy lifestyle

by Dr Peter W. Bennett, co-author of *The 7 day-detox miracle*.

As a naturopathic physician, I have been treating patients with detoxification strategies for 20 years. I use detoxification methods because they bring results. Often I will see immediate results in healthy people who just want more energy, want to lose some weight or want to renew their minds and spirits.

I am firmly convinced that detoxification and purification are important strategies we should all use to boost our health and promote healing. Purification and medical detoxification are so effective because they stimulate the body's own healing mechanisms and enhance the body's ability to filter and clean the blood. By resting the immune and detoxification organs of the digestive tract and promoting elimination, we can recharge our body's ability to heal.

There is a rich heritage in the history of medicine for the use of detoxification medicine. Going back to Hippocrates, fasting, diet therapy and hydrotherapy have been used with great effect to successfully treat a wide range of health disorders. Even with the recent advancements in biochemistry, physiology and pharmacology, the ancient wisdom of detoxification therapy in maintaining health and curing a wide range of disease processes remains unequalled.

Yet even now, despite valid clinical results across the world, detoxification techniques are little understood and still underprescribed in the medical treatment of chronic conditions like asthma, heart disease, migraines and fatigue.

That's why the editors of Rodale Health Books have done such a great service to readers in bringing together this vast assortment of purification and detoxification techniques in *Detox!* With the practical details provided in this book, you can gain immense benefits from adopting purification methods in your own self care. Through a detoxifying diet you can boost your immunity to disease. With the use of safe and effective herbs you can improve digestion and fight infection.

Healing exercises and meditation can help to stimulate your circulatory and nervous systems to keep stress from poisoning your body. You'll also be introduced to the world of more intensive, professional detoxification methods like panchakarma and lymphatic drainage massage to help you to decide whether they offer the healing you seek.

In addition to describing the immediate health benefits that these purification methods can bring you, this book offers the hope that you will be able to protect yourself and your family from the scourge of everyday toxins in your life. You will find safe, simple, yet powerful ways to reverse the damage and smart advice on reducing or preventing further exposure.

In some ways, modern medicine is like the Titanic. You'll remember that even though the crew could see the iceberg ahead, they could not turn the ship fast enough to protect its passengers. Modern medicine knows about the negative impact of pollution, toxins, dysbiosis, heavy metals and stress hormones, but it cannot provide a drug or surgical therapy to deal with such a complex mess of problems facing society.

But now, in the pages of *Detox!*, you have at your disposal some of the most effective healing methods ever developed. When you use these purification strategies in your life, every day will be a little farther down the road to happiness and healing.

How to use this book

You are about to discover techniques that range from simple recipes and exercise advice to herbal remedies and professional treatments developed from ancient healing practices – all brought together in one place and explained for maximum safety and effectiveness.

The first section of the book will help you to understand why detoxification is so critical to restoring and maintaining your health and vitality. You will learn the practical strategies that you can use in your path to better health. For each of the primary means of detoxification, you will find information on how to employ what are familiar aspects of healthy living in remarkable new ways. The result will be to purify your body and build immunity to the toxins you encounter at home, at work and in the environment. With these secrets, you can unlock the full promise of better health and healing by applying the purifying power of food, herbs, exercise, fasting and cleansing, emotional healing, home spa treatments and professional therapies.

In the second section of the book, you'll discover the strategy that makes it so easy to make detoxification a part of your healthy lifestyle. The strategy starts with a general-purpose 7-day plan that is a great place for virtually everyone to begin on the path of purification. This is followed by chapters on exercise, recipes and home treatments. You'll then find targeted plans and tips for specific conditions that may be of particular concern for you. In all, more than 50 specific health problems are addressed. The plan concludes with hints and tips for 'staying clean'. Chapter 15 contains safe and easy ways to avoid toxic exposure and keep your newly purified body in a fully functioning state of health.

Your strategy for putting *Detox!* into action can be as simple as 1-2-3.

1 **Try the 7-day *Detox!* plan** to begin to reverse the toxic build-up in your body.

2 **Choose a targeted detoxification** for a condition that concerns you, or build on the 7-day plan using your preferred methods of general detoxification such as healing foods, herbs, fasting, cleansing, exercise or spa treatments.

3 **Reduce your exposure to more toxins** by following the advice in Chapter 15, Staying Clean: 34 steps to toxin-free living.

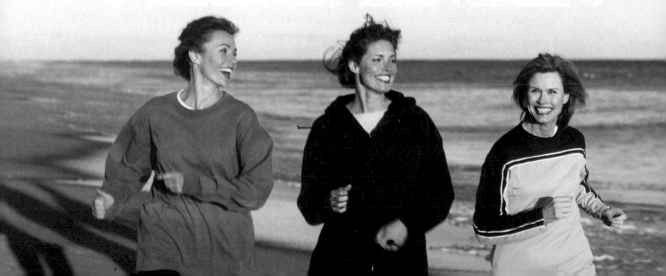

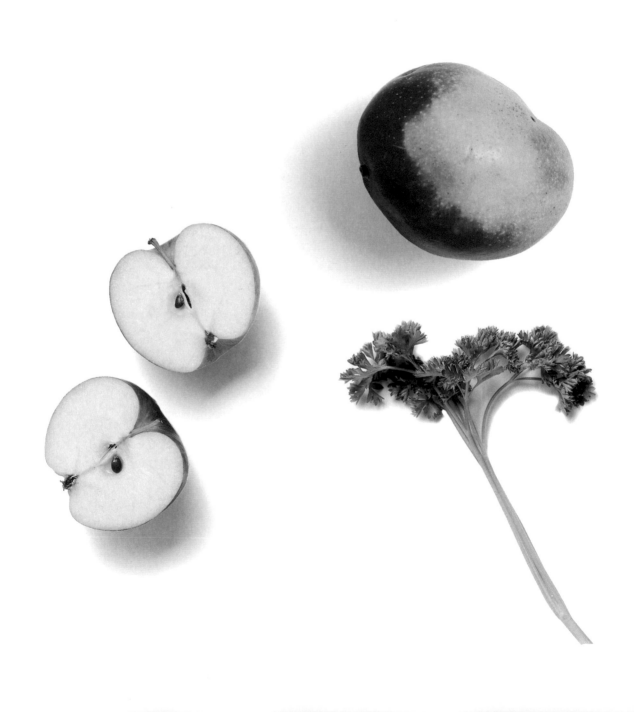

Detox!

Understanding what your body needs

There are many paths to healing,
but all paths share one common goal:
to restore your body's natural ability to heal itself.
In this section, you'll discover the remarkable
capacity that detoxification has to provide the
restorative balance that your body needs.
What's more, you'll learn the secrets of the safest,
most effective purification methods you can use in
your own home. From familiar remedies like
healing foods, herbs and exercise, to fasting and
relaxing therapeutic spa treatments, you'll be able
to find the paths to healing that best suit your
health needs and lifestyle.

Chapter 1
Healing with detoxification
Why your body needs a little help

Your body cleans itself all the time and it's all the more amazing because it happens automatically. If you were to concentrate on the detoxification work that goes on continuously in your body, you'd probably never get anything else done.

Your liver, for example, is going to clean your blood of toxins whether you tell it to or not. But if you overload your liver's ability to detoxify your body, you run the risk of compromising the organ that helps to keep you from getting cancer. So it's a good idea to do what you can to avoid exposure to toxins whenever you can. It's also a good idea to increase your body's ability to detoxify itself in every way that you can. These two goals are what this book is all about.

Let's take a brief look at how the self-cleaning actions of your body's systems work. Then we'll look at the toxic challenges that your body comes up against on a daily basis.

Facing the toxic onslaught

Toxins are in the air you breathe, the water you drink, the food you eat, your household cleaners and body-care products, your child's plastic toys

THE BODY'S FIVE CLEANSING ORGANS

Five specific organs play critical roles in helping to escort toxins from your body. They're known as the organs of elimination.

• Your liver filters toxins from your blood, removing bacteria, viruses and environmental pollutants such as pesticides, drugs, and household and industrial chemicals.

• The lungs take in oxygen and get rid of volatile gases and carbon dioxide. Your lungs also produce mucus, to trap toxins and impurities so that they can be coughed out.

• The kidneys process about 200 litres (44 gallons) of blood every day to sift out about 2 litres (3½ pints) of waste products and extra water, which come from the normal breakdown of active tissues and from food. The waste and extra water become urine.

• The skin is covered by sweat glands that eliminate waste – primarily urea and ammonia – in the form of perspiration.

• The intestines absorb nutrients from the food you eat. The remains enter your large intestine, called the colon, which absorbs needed water and minerals and transports waste to the rectum for elimination.

and your freshly dry-cleaned clothing. And they're in you. Your body generates them as it carries out its normal functions – breathing, eating, even going for your daily walk.

NO ONE IS IMMUNE

Science has linked manufactured toxins in the environment to a wide variety of chronic degenerative diseases such as asthma, Alzheimer's disease, cancer and coronary artery disease, to name just a few. But some studies have associated these substances with specific conditions that affect men, women and children. The table below lists some of these.

Women
- Breast, ovarian and uterine cancers
- Endometriosis
- Infertility and sterility
- Miscarriage
- Premenstrual syndrome (PMS)
- Uterine fibroids

Children*
- Attention Deficit Disorder
- Attention Deficit Hyperactivity Disorder
- Autism
- Birth defects of the penis and testicles in boys
- Childhood cancers, including brain tumours and leukaemia
- Early puberty in girls (increases risk of breast cancer in adulthood)

Men
- Decreased fertility and sterility
- Diminished sperm count
- Testicular cancer

*Certain forms of childhood cancer have been linked to exposure by parent or child to toxic chemicals such as pesticides.

Your body also carries a burden of 'emotional toxins' such as stress, anger and depression. They affect the ways in which you think and feel, and how you process environmental toxins.

If the body can't rid itself of toxins, they back up in the blood, cells and tissues, causing a kind of low-grade poisoning. The weaker the body's ability to cleanse itself, the more vulnerable to illness it is. There's a lot you can do to build up your body's ability to eliminate the internal and external poisons that threaten it. The key is taking charge of your health. You have to educate yourself about environmental toxins and how they can affect your health.

While there's no way you can avoid all the toxins coming at you, you can take steps to avoid unnecessary exposure to a great many. There are also strategies that you can incorporate into your life to help to support your body's efforts to throw off any toxins that do make it into your body. In this book you'll find out how to customize a purification plan to meet your personal needs.

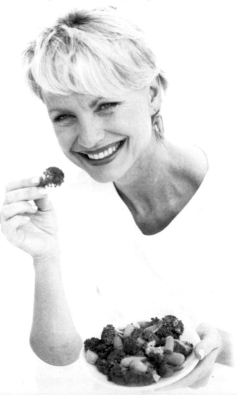

The toxins we must all deal with are categorized by their effects on human health:

Carcinogens cause genetic alterations that lead to cancerous tumours or promote the growth of cancer cells.

Developmental toxins harm a foetus in the womb, causing birth defects or behavioural problems.

Reproductive toxins damage the male and female reproductive systems, which can cause infertility.

Endocrine disrupters affect the functioning of hormones, including the female sex hormone oestrogen, raising the risk of hormone-fuelled cancers such as breast cancer.

Phthalates are used to manufacture countless household items, from toys and shower curtains to nail polish and wallpaper. These chemicals have been linked to birth defects, liver and thyroid damage, a decline in the quantity and quality of sperm in men and miscarriages in women. At least one phthalate, Di(2-ethylhexyl) phthalate (DEHP), is likely to cause cancer.

Volatile organic compounds (VOCs) – a class of substances widely used in industry and manufacturing and found in household products such as cleansers, aerosol sprays, air fresheners and dry-cleaned clothing – are a significant source of our body burden. These include solvents, which are substances used to dissolve other substances and which are found in paint, paint strippers and petrol. Solvents are toxic to both the nervous system and immune systems. They have been linked to brain tumours and leukaemia in children.

Immunotoxic chemicals interfere with or damage the body's immune system.

Having a 'bad air day'?

While some air toxins come from natural sources, such as forest fires, most are manufactured. These include benzene, found in fuel; perchloro-ethylene, used in dry cleaning; and methylene chloride, an industrial solvent.

Then there are dioxins, the by-products of burning wastes and chemical manufacturing. Considered to be some of the most toxic chemicals known, dioxins don't dissolve in water, but they do dissolve in fat – our fat. They're hard to get rid of, once absorbed.

And there's acid rain. When fuels such as coal and oil are burned at high temperatures, they form gases called nitrogen oxides and sulphur dioxide. These gases interact in the atmosphere and fall in the form of rain, snow and fog. When they evaporate, they form dry gases and particles that are transported by winds and inhaled by us.

These toxic air pollutants have been linked to cancer, reduced fertility, birth defects, and heart and lung problems. Studies suggest that diesel exhaust doesn't just aggravate asthma, it may cause it. The fine particles in diesel exhaust may cause alterations in the immune system which may cause asthma in otherwise healthy people.

But you don't just breathe in air toxins. They can also get into water and soil, which means that you can absorb them by drinking water polluted by these chemicals; eating fish from polluted waters or meat, milk or eggs from animals that were fed on contaminated plants; or eating fruits and vegetables grown in soil in which these toxins have been deposited. Children can absorb them when they place their soil-covered hands or toys in their mouths.

However, it is possible to avoid some of these toxins by paying careful attention to the sources of the foods you eat, and by making careful choices about the kinds of products you use in your home. Even though you've undoubtedly been exposed to many of these toxins and have some stored in your tissues, you don't need to carry them around with you forever. Throughout this book you'll find remedies using herbs, foods and even spa treatments that will help to enhance the ongoing cleansing process that lessens your body's burden.

Toxins on tap

The water we drink looks clean but it may contain more than 2,000 toxic chemicals, including industrial chemicals, pesticides and toxic metals.

Lead is one of the most pervasive contaminants in drinking water. Typically, the lead isn't in the water itself, but in lead pipes, joints and solder, usually found in very old homes. Babies and children who drink lead-tainted water may suffer physical and developmental delays. Adults who drink it over many years can develop kidney problems or high blood pressure.

Outdated treatment plants also threaten our drinking water. Treatment plants were designed to remove organic wastes such as bacteria, not man-made chemicals. So when this chemical-laced water passes through the treatment plant, the chemicals remain.

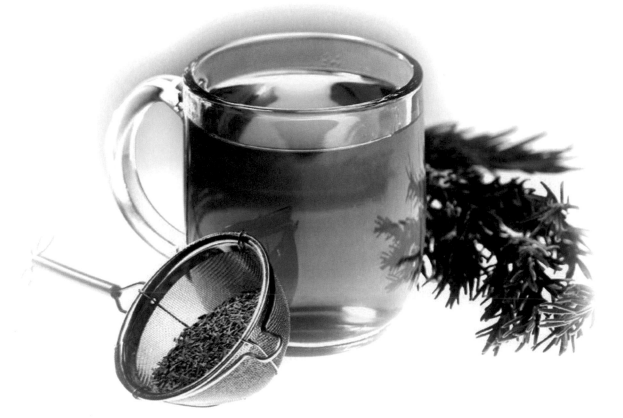

A plateful of poisons

No matter how wholesome the food you eat appears to be, the chances are that you're also ingesting a chemical stew of pesticides (used to prevent crop damage by weeds, insects, rodents and moulds) or other dangerous substances.

The meat and milk we eat and drink are laced with chemicals such as growth hormones and antibiotics, as well.

A junk-food diet is also toxic to the body. It's high in calories and refined carbohydrates, like white flour and white sugar, and low in vitamins, minerals and phytonutrients – the good-for-you substances in fruits, vegetables and whole grains shown to reduce the risk of cancer and other degenerative diseases.

Processed foods such as salty snack foods and sweet biscuits contain trans fatty acids, now known to be as unhealthy for your heart as the saturated fat in bacon and butter. (Some food manufacturers now reveal the amount of trans and unsaturated fats in their products.) Chemicals added to food to preserve its freshness or add flavour can also 'poison' the body.

CHILDREN ARE MOST AT RISK

There's growing evidence that children are most susceptible to environmental toxins. Pound for pound, children eat, drink and breathe more than adults, which means that they absorb proportionally larger doses of toxins. Children also have faster metabolisms, which speeds up their absorption of these chemicals. For example, children absorb about 50 percent of the lead they swallow, while adults absorb about 10 percent. Plus, they play on the floor, where the highest concentrations of pollutants settle.

While you can't hope to eliminate all the toxins from your food, the food choices you make every day are among your most important tools for detoxification. You'll find a variety of suggestions for boosting your energy and preventing disease in Chapter 3.

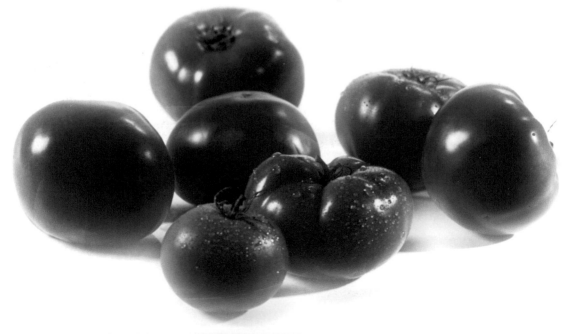

Home, toxic home

People tend to be most concerned about outdoor air pollution, but indoor air is much more toxic than the air outside. In fact, concentrations of volatile organic compounds (VOCs) are two to five times higher inside our homes than they are outdoors. And don't forget about cigarette smoke, perhaps the deadliest household toxin. Passive smoking causes about 17,000 deaths in the UK every year and smoking-related illnesses account for 8 million visits to the doctor annually.

The very materials used to build your home may contain health-threatening chemicals. For example, the formaldehyde used in furniture (especially if MDF is used) and decorative wall coverings can sting your eyes and throat, make you feel queasy and make it difficult to breathe. It may also cause cancer.

Asbestos, a mineral fibre used for insulation, has been shown to cause lung cancer. While asbestos is no longer used, older homes may have it in ductwork, pipe wraps or other materials, and removing it improperly can cause its fibres to be released into the air and inhaled.

Perchloroethylene, commonly used in dry cleaning, has been shown to cause cancer in animals. Research shows that people breathe low levels of this chemical at home, where their dry-cleaned clothing is stored.

Work is no less toxic. An investigation conducted in 2000 by the newspaper *USA Today* found that employees in more than 35 states unknowingly carried toxins from work to home in their cars and on their shoes, clothes, hair, tools and briefcases, potentially exposing their families to mercury, radioactive material, lead, asbestos, PCBs and pesticides.

Office workers are frequently trapped in office buildings with windows that don't open and inhale fumes emitted by plastic chairs, new carpets and MDF particleboard.

Solvents, paints or other chemicals can be absorbed on-the-job either by direct contact or by the fumes being inhaled. Unfortunately, chemical sensitivity is usually only discovered after people have become sick.

Body-care products are another source of potentially toxic chemicals. Because makeup is not considered a food or drug, it is not regulated for the safety of its ingredients. But some cosmetics contain nitrosamines, which have been found to cause cancer.

Talc is a mineral commonly used in powders and other makeup. A study in Seattle found that women with ovarian cancer are more likely to have used powder products and sprays in the genital area than women without the disease. It may also impair fertility.

For a good, overall look at how to select body-care products and use them wisely, see Chapter 12.

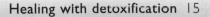

Chapter 2
Detoxification partners
Safe and effective ways to detox

Imagine yourself more energetic, better able to reduce your medications, shrug off stress and fatigue and set yourself free from aches, pains, sneezes and sniffles. In short, imagine looking and feeling better than you have for years.

Detoxification can help you to reap all of these benefits and more. Practised for centuries by cultures around the world, detoxification is the process of eliminating the body's 'toxic build-up', helping it to repair and renew itself.

The body has its own natural healing system, and detoxification rejuvenates the body's natural ability to cleanse itself of waste generated by cells and tissues as they do their work, as well as man-made chemicals in air, water and food.

Detoxification is now more important than ever; in addition to the health problems we've experienced for thousands of years, we are now exposed to a huge variety of environmental poisons. Detoxification can ease your body's toxic burden because not only does it help to eliminate the toxins already in your body but it minimizes the absorption of new ones.

Detoxification isn't a New Age fad. Although it has taken many forms, detoxifying the body is a serious healing concept practised for centuries in cultures around the world. For example, Native Americans use sweat lodges to purify and renew their bodies and spirits, and Scandinavians prescribe the sauna for their ills. Practitioners of ayurveda, the ancient system of medicine in India, view many diseases as the accumulation of toxic materials in the digestive system, and recommend fasting.

Today, more and more people are discovering detoxification's rejuvenating powers. Alternative practitioners contend that, properly used, a number of detoxification practices can strengthen the body's immune system, as well as the 'purification system', which is made up of the liver, kidneys and other organs. Without having to carry its toxic burden, the body is better able to repair itself and stay at peak health.

Purification should be an ongoing process. Still, it's wise to undergo a more formal cleansing at least once a year. You can certainly detoxify more often than that, if you wish. Of course there are exceptions: pregnant women, nursing mothers, children and people with cancer, as well as people who have low body weight, psychiatric illness or other serious diseases. Anyone in doubt should consult a doctor.

There are many purification methods, all of which can be used alone or in combination. The following are the techniques most commonly used by alternative practitioners.

Healing diet

A diet of whole, organic, natural foods gives the body the nutrients it needs to nourish cells and tissues and cleanse stored poisons from the colon (large intestine) and other organs. It also gives your intestinal tract a break from the white flour, white sugar and artery-clogging fats as well as the caffeine and alcohol in the typical Western diet.

How a healing diet works

A detoxifying diet helps your body to release substances that it might otherwise struggle to release, thereby relieving poor digestion, headaches, fatigue, joint pain and other symptoms. It includes fresh fruits and vegetables and whole grains that contain fibre, which helps your colon to eliminate toxins.

Ideally, a detoxifying diet is something that you do for a lifetime. However, it is possible to follow a stricter form of eating for a short period of time and experience considerable benefits. This kind of diet is typically paired with herbs and supplements known to eliminate toxins. Most alternative practitioners recommend following a strict one to two-week detoxification diet twice yearly.

Benefits

When you give your body a break from the toxins in your diet, even for as little as a few days, you can shed excess water weight, boost your energy and mood, and lose that vaguely sick, bloated feeling. Even mild changes from your current way of eating will produce some benefits, while more dramatic changes over a long period can produce a profound improvement in health.

Drawbacks

Some people may experience headaches and fatigue for the first few days of a detox diet. This is normal as the body releases toxins. These symptoms usually fade by the third or fourth day. And if you are not used to eating a lot of fibre you may experience wind and abdominal discomfort.

A healing diet works best for:

Men and women in good general health. Although children should generally not be put on a strict 'cleansing diet', they can benefit from following it in a milder form. That is, they should eat lots of fresh fruits and vegetables and whole grains, and fewer (or no) processed junk foods.

ARE YOU HAVING A HEALING CRISIS?

You've cleaned up your diet, stopped smoking and started taking a brisk walk each day. You're feeling great and then, out of nowhere, you're hit with fatigue, headaches, and an all-over ill feeling. What's happening? You are probably in the midst of what alternative practitioners call a healing crisis – a temporary surge in symptoms that often occurs during the purification process. Believe it or not, a healing crisis signals that the body is on the mend.

Here's what happens: as your body begins to purify itself and get healthier, it begins to eliminate toxic residues that it has stored for a long time, sometimes for years. These residues include traces of old chemicals stored in fat tissue, remnants of prescription medications from your blood, and other wastes. This surge of toxins causes symptoms that may include constipation or diarrhoea, headaches, nausea, and sores or skin problems. You may feel better for a day or two, suddenly feel worse again, and then feel better again.

One healing crisis may not purge all of the toxins that have built up in your body over the years, but each successive crisis will become milder and of shorter duration. To help to minimize the healing crisis, get lots of rest, drink plenty of water and reduce stress as much as possible. If the symptoms don't pass after three or four days, however, consult your doctor. It can be difficult to determine the difference between a healing crisis and an illness.

Healing herbs

Herbs have a long medical tradition. For example, herbal remedies are in the *Papyrus Ebers*, a medical guide used by doctors in ancient Egypt. Thousands of years later, alternative practitioners still use specific herbs to support detoxification and promote healing.

How healing herbs work

There are two main classes of detoxification herbs. The first class of herbs, the 'housekeeping' herbs, speeds toxins out of the body by increasing production of urine, sweat and bile (an enzyme, produced by the liver, that aids digestion) or by revving up immune cells.

The second class of herbs, known as adaptogens, raises the body's resistance to toxins, as well as physical and emotional stresses. You'll learn more about these herbs in Chapter 4.

Benefits

Herbs are available in almost any form, including fresh (ready to add to cooking), easy-to-swallow capsules, tablets, liquid drops (tinctures), and teas made from fresh or dried herbs. Most such herbs are non-toxic and are not habit-forming.

Drawbacks

Herbs don't normally work quickly. They may take weeks or even months to work, so be patient. Some herbs may also cause minor side effects, especially when used in combination with prescription or over-the-counter drugs, or when used by people with pre-existing health conditions.

Healing herbs work best for:

Healthy adult men and women. Unless you're working with a health care professional who is experienced in prescribing herbs, don't take herbs if you're pregnant or have kidney disease, high blood pressure, diabetes or any other serious health condition. While certain herbs are safe for children, they should not be given herbs with a powerful laxative effect. Let a naturopathic health care professional work with them; their needs are special and require extra training.

Exercise

Regular exercise is essential to the purification process. While any sweat-inducing physical activity will aid the body's detoxification efforts, three types – yoga, tai chi and qi gong – are particularly associated with purification.

How exercise works

Regular exercise boosts your circulation of blood and lymph, the fluid produced by your lymph system. Improved circulation carries nutrients, oxygen and immune cells to damaged cells or tissues and carries away cellular waste and other toxins. Physical activity also promotes sweating, which eliminates toxins through the skin, and increases the frequency of bowel movements.

Even moderate exercise on a regular basis helps to melt excess body fat. Since fat is a primary storage site for toxins, getting rid of excess body fat is an important part of detoxification.

Benefits

The benefits of yoga for detoxification are unequalled. It encourages the proper circulation of blood and lymph fluid, enhances digestion and lubricates the joints, among other benefits.

Moderate exercise boosts the body's immune system, which can help the body to resist the effects of environmental toxins. For example, regular brisk walking has been shown to bolster specific aspects of the immune system, including cancer-fighting natural killer (NK) cells. Being active also reduces your risk of degenerative diseases, including heart disease, high blood pressure and diabetes, improves flexibility and sleep and relieves stress.

Drawbacks

While moderately intensive exercise helps to eliminate toxins, too much exercise can actually weaken the immune system because during intense physical exertion, the body produces cortisol and adrenaline, stress hormones that temporarily suppress the immune system.

Exercise works best for:

Almost everyone. Government guidelines call for adults and older people to engage in moderate physical activity five or more times a week for at least 30 minutes at a time. Children need at least an hour of moderate activity most days of the week. If you are over 50 or have health issues, get your doctor's approval before you embark on an exercise programme. For more information on safe and healthy exercise as part of your detoxification efforts, see Chapter 5.

Fasting

Fasting – going without solid food for a day or longer – is one of the oldest therapeutic practices in medicine. While the most stringent form of fasting allows the intake of only water, most alternative practitioners recommend juice fasts, featuring the freshly made juices of a variety of fruits and vegetables.

Unlike water alone, fresh juices supply nutrients the body needs to help to eliminate toxins and rejuvenate cells and tissues.

How fasting works

The typical juice fast consists of drinking 2 to 3 litres (3½ to 5 pints) of water and freshly squeezed fruit and vegetable juices over the course of a day. Fruits are considered the best purifiers, and vegetables the best cellular rebuilders.

Ideally, the fruits and vegetables you juice should be organic. If organic produce isn't available, fruits and vegetables should be thoroughly washed and peeled.

During a fast, the cells in your body begin to release stored fat. When this fat is burned, the toxins within it are released and eventually eliminated from the body.

Experts recommend that beginners start with a one-day fast before attempting something longer. They also recommend that several days before beginning a fast, you should start preparing your body by eliminating caffeine, nicotine, alcohol and animal foods from your diet and eat only fruits and vegetables.

Benefits

A juice fast allows many of the body's systems a rest. Cells have the opportunity to repair themselves and eliminate their waste, and the liver can spend more time on the important process of detoxification. Fasting is also a good way to break bad eating habits.

Drawbacks

If you don't already have a juicer, try to find a fairly basic one that will meet your needs without being too expensive or too complicated to use.

During a fast, you may experience unpleasant symptoms, such as weakness, headaches, fatigue and dizziness. However, these symptoms usually pass in two or three days and, if you do a shorter fast or a modified fast, you may not experience any.

Fasts that consist only of water can actually hinder the process of detoxification if done for a few days. That's because water-only fasts deplete the body of nutrients critical to the detoxification process, such as antioxidant vitamins and the enzyme glutathione. They also lack protein – which the liver uses to detoxify – and fibre, which sweeps the digestive tract clean, escorting toxins out of the body.

It is possible to benefit from longer, water-only fasts, but these must be done only under the supervision of a health care professional experienced in supervising therapeutic fasts.

Fasting works best for:

Adult men and women in good health. Do not fast if you're pregnant or nursing, if you're underweight, or if you have recently had or will soon have surgery. People with chronic health problems such as cancer or heart disease should fast only under the supervision of a doctor experienced in using fasts as therapy. Children should not fast.

THE BENEFITS OF EMOTIONAL DETOX

Detoxification doesn't just benefit your body; it can also increase your emotional well-being. Similarly, neutralizing emotional 'toxins' such as anger and depression can reduce your body's vulnerability to physical ills.

Cleansing your mind and spirit of past hurts and resentments is just as important as cleansing your body of toxins. Emotionally, detoxification helps us to uncover and express feelings, especially hidden frustrations, anger, resentments or fear, and replace them with forgiveness, love, joy and hope.

On a spiritual level, many people experience new clarity and/or an enhancement of their purpose in life during cleansing processes. When your body has eliminated much of its toxic build-up, you feel lighter and are able to really experience the moment and be open to the future.

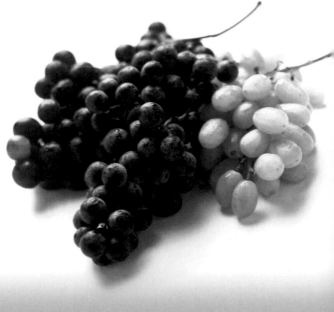

Colonic cleansing

As far back as the ancient Egyptians, enemas were commonly used to cleanse the colon and rid the body of toxins believed to cause ill health. Practitioners believe that over time, undigested food and faecal waste harden and accumulate on the walls of the bowels, hindering the bowels' attempts to eliminate it. These materials decay and are thought to lead to a host of symptoms that range from frequent headaches to overall ill health.

How cleansing works

There are three main ways to cleanse: natural laxatives, enemas and colonics. An enema is a self-administered injection of warm, distilled water into the colon by way of a tube inserted into the rectum. It cleanses the lower portion of the large intestine and uses about 2 litres (3½ pints) of liquid.

A colonic is a more extensive cleansing technique, which uses 90 or more litres (20 gallons) of water to cleanse the colon's entire 4.5m (15ft) length. It requires the use of a special machine that pumps the water into the bowel with a hose and then drains the waste. In either method, the water loosens waste in the colon so it can be eliminated through the rectum.

Benefits

Flushing out impacted faecal matter, toxins, mucus and parasites from the intestines eliminates the toxic build-up that may cause ill health and disease. Cleansing also boosts the transit of matter through the bowel allowing it to better absorb nutrients from food, which can help to improve the symptoms of vitamin and other nutrient deficiencies. Many people with intestinal problems or chronic headaches say they experience almost immediate relief after colonic cleansing.

A FRAGRANT WAY TO CLEANSE THE SPIRIT

Aromatherapy has been used to increase physical and emotional well-being since the time of the ancient Egyptians. This therapy's uses include relieving pain, nausea, colds, skin problems and other conditions. Its stress-relieving qualities are also used in detoxification.

Aromatherapy uses the essential oils of plants, which have been chemically extracted from aromatic flowers, herbs and even woods. Each essential oil has its own characteristic aroma and therapeutic effects. There are oils to soothe, to invigorate and to relieve negative emotions, such as depression, stress and anxiety. Still other essential oils are believed to battle bacteria and fungi and reduce inflammation.

Essential oils are used in many different ways, including massage, inhalation, aromatic baths, compresses and vaporization. Some of the oils commonly used for detoxification purposes include angelica root, fennel, grapefruit and juniper berry.

Essential oils are very concentrated, so never apply them directly to your skin. Before you use them, you must dilute them in a pure, natural 'carrier' oil, such as sweet almond oil, apricot oil or grape seed oil.

Aromatherapy isn't for everyone, however. Avoid it if you have asthma, high blood pressure, cancer, sensitive skin or allergies, or if you are pregnant. Also, avoid using essential oils on babies and children. And never, ever take it orally.

Drawbacks

Some people may find colonic cleansing to be physically or mentally unpleasant. While many people are used to taking gentle, natural laxatives, enemas and colonics require time and a matter-of-fact attitude.

Cleansing works best for:

People who suffer from chronic constipation and stress, or are overweight. These conditions tend to make the bowels sluggish and hinder digestion. Don't cleanse if you have a gastrointestinal condition such as Crohn's disease or diverticulitis, or a serious condition such as heart disease or high blood pressure. If you opt for a colonic, make sure it's performed by a qualified practitioner.

For more information on fasting and cleansing, see Chapter 6.

Hydrotherapy

The practice of using water to promote healing, hydrotherapy has been part of the healing tradition of almost every civilization and is a cornerstone of detoxification therapy.

How hydrotherapy works

Hydrotherapy consists of using hot and cold water in various ways to improve circulation and stimulate the immune system. Methods include hot and cold baths and showers, steam and sauna therapy, and constitutional hydrotherapy, in which alternating hot and cold packs are placed on the body, front and back.

Benefits

Hydrotherapy intensifies blood circulation to the liver, kidneys and intestines, which helps these organs excrete waste. In steam and sauna therapy, toxins from the bloodstream are eliminated through the skin via sweat.

Drawbacks

Some forms of hydrotherapy can be time-consuming and, for some people, uncomfortable. For example, the wet-sheet method calls for lying in a tub filled with water as hot as possible, then quickly wrapping up in a cold, wet sheet. Also, excessively hot or cold water applied directly to the skin for long periods may cause discomfort or even tissue damage.

Hydrotherapy works best for:

Healthy men and women. However, sauna therapy is not for everyone. Avoid these techniques if you are pregnant or have a serious health problem such as diabetes, high blood pressure, heart disease or a seizure disorder. And sauna therapy should not be used by children – they can become dangerously dehydrated.

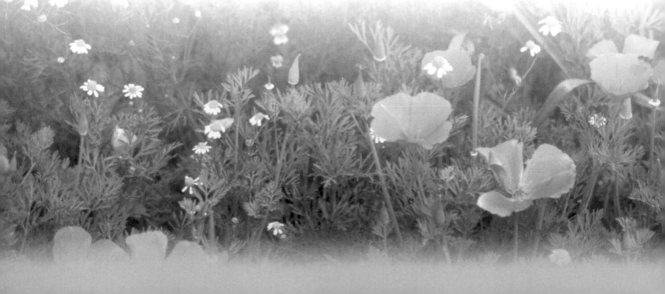

Chapter 3
The essential foods
Choosing a diet for detoxification

If you've been eating healthily to prevent disease, boost your energy, keep your weight down and remain youthful as long as possible, then you will already have come across the rules in this chapter.

The following statements will probably sound familiar to you. Rather than quick fixes, they offer a long-term change in your approach to eating that can dramatically improve your health.

- Consume a wide variety of whole grains, fruits, and vegetables, preferably organic.
- Stay away from processed foods, fatty foods – except oily fish – hydrogenated oils, food additives and sugar.
- Drink plenty of pure, clean water.

These rules are also what it takes to not only detoxify your body, but to keep it clean inside once you've rid yourself of the toxins. In fact, almost every health care professional who places emphasis on detoxifying the body as a means to a longer, healthier life, emphasizes the importance of eating the right kinds of foods on a regular basis.

'I'd rather clean my house all the time than give it a really good cleaning once a year,' says Suzzanne Myer MS, RD, of the nutrition faculty at Bastyr Center for Natural Health in Seattle. By 'cleaning my house all the time', she means eating the foods that keep her system clean.

'The bottom line is that I eat from the earth to me, whole grains, fruits, vegetables, eggs, dairy,' says Carrie Demers MD, director of the Himalayan Institute's Center for Health and Healing in Pennsylvania. In her own life, she says, she concentrates on 'food that's really fresh and whole, food that's rich in life force – prana. (*Prana*, the

Sanskrit word for life force or life energy, is a concept that has become widespread as untold thousands of people worldwide turn to yoga as their exercise of choice.) 'If you don't do anything else,' advises Dr Demers, 'add more fresh food to your diet. Those fresh foods have fibre.'

It is interesting how many health care professionals from different fields of study refer to the need to 'eat close to the earth' when talking about how to eat correctly, detoxify and keep the body clean.

What is it about this kind of eating that helps the body to purify itself?

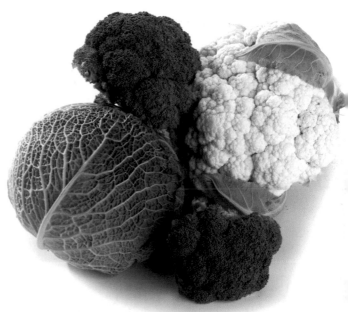

To help you to understand how foods that are 'close to the Earth' actually make a difference, we'll look at the liver, because that's one of the body's main detoxifying organs, and the same foods that support the liver support the other organs and cleansing systems as well.

Fibre power

There is no doubt that your liver is perhaps your body's best filter of toxins. It's where everything from caffeine and alcohol to pesticide residues, heavy metals and prescription medications gets filtered out of your body. But you may not realize that by eating a high-fibre diet, you can actually help this filter to do its job better.

As part of the digestion process, your liver manufactures bile salts, substances made partly from cholesterol. Bile gets squirted into your gallbladder, where it's stored until you eat something. Then it gets squirted into your small intestine to help your body to digest fats. The liver uses the bile as a run-off place for toxins – just one of the places it stores toxins. Under ideal conditions, the bile does its job of helping to digest fats and then most of it gets swept from the body along with the waste products of digestion.

'Ideal conditions' are when you eat a natural diet high in fibre, and then form a good bulky stool, the soluble fibre binding up the bile salts and moving it through your body swiftly. The remains of a meal eaten one day should come out the other end in 24 hours or less.

But if you don't eat a high-fibre diet – let's say you eat the stereotypical meat-and-potatoes-white-bread diet, instead – it will take a lot longer for a stool to move through your body – two to three days or even longer. And since your liver is an efficient machine, it can reuse bile salts. Instead of some of the bile salts sliding out of your body the way nature intended, most gets reabsorbed, moving back to your liver and getting used again the next time you eat a fatty meal.

The problem here is that your liver uses cholesterol to make bile salts. So if it doesn't need to make new bile salts, some cholesterol that you could have got rid of will stay in your blood. And if your liver has stored some toxins in that bile, you may reabsorb them back into your body.

Your best sources of fibre are whole grains, fruits and vegetables. There are all kinds of ways to add considerably to the fibre you're already taking in.

Double your oat power If you enjoy oatmeal for breakfast, increase its fibre power by stirring in a tablespoon of oat bran. You won't taste the difference, but you've just added a little more scrubbing power to your body's cleansing system. Actually, you can add oat bran to any hot cereal, as well as to chilli and meat loaf.

Try some apple slices Before you sit down in front of the TV for the evening, peel and core an apple. Cut it into thin slices and put them in a bowl. Add a bowl of chunky peanut butter for dipping. Or you could try some raisins or other fruit.

Bring it with you Packing an orange or a peach or a little bag of sliced carrots along with those lunchtime sandwiches is always a good idea. This will help you to spread your fibre consumption out over the entire day, too, rather than eating a whole day's worth at one sitting.

Put beans in your salads Open and rinse a can of kidney beans or chickpeas and throw a couple of handfuls into your salad. You can even do this with prepared salads picked up on the way home from work. It's a good way to make a 'low-calorie, light bite' feel like a really substantial meal. Salads already pack a high-fibre wallop. Half a cup of canned kidney beans has 7.9 grams (¼ oz) of fibre; a half-cup of canned chickpeas has 7 grams (¼ oz). That's a lot of fibre in just a little bit of food.

Pop your own In place of potato crisps (minimal fibre), put out bowls of air-popped popcorn. It's a low-calorie snack that satisfies your appetite and bumps up fibre intake.

Bump it up slowly If you and your family aren't used to getting a lot of extra fibre, you might want to ease into it slowly. If you eat too much, too quickly, you could experience bloating, abdominal discomfort and wind. If you gradually increase the amount of fibre you eat, your body will take it in its stride and you should suffer none of the unpleasant side effects.

Wash it down If you eat a lot of fibre, you also need to drink plenty of water to keep things moving. You should drink at least eight 225ml (8fl oz) glasses a day. Young children, of course, can drink less, but they still need to drink three or four glasses of water a day.

Of course, you can always take a fibre supplement, and that might be a good idea if you're also dealing with high cholesterol. But there are some really good reasons why you should get your key nutrients from food.

TWO-STAGE CLEANSING POWER

Researchers have found that the liver does its detoxification work in two main phases.

• During the first stage, a set of enzymes known as cytochrome p450 transforms toxic substances into intermediate chemicals.

• Then the second stage of detoxification, which takes place in several steps, turns those intermediate chemicals into water-soluble substances that can be flushed from the body.

Sometimes our poor liver is detoxifying things it's never experienced before in our chemical world. It gets through phase one, then doesn't know what to do with the substances. That can slow things down. One challenge that your body is faced with is that these intermediate chemicals are frequently even more toxic than the chemicals that you're trying to get rid of in the first place. If the second stage of your liver's detox system is not adequately supported by good nutrition, your body has to deal with serious toxic build-up.

Nutrients for filtering power

The liver uses some 50 to 100 separate enzymes to filter and detoxify food wastes, pesticide residues, alcohol and other poisons that get into your blood. That means your liver needs literally dozens of separate chemicals in order to do its job correctly and keep your body toxin-free and healthy. And all of these biochemicals – or the components to manufacture them – must come from the foods that you eat on a regular basis.

There's no way that you could take a couple of supplements and cover all your bases. That's one of the reasons that health care professionals point to a nature-based diet, rather than supplements, as a way to be sure of meeting your needs.

However, they do recommend taking a good multivitamin supplement as insurance that you're getting at least some of what you need. And if you are being seen by an experienced health care practitioner, you might be prescribed some additional supplements to meet your individual needs. But all experts on nutrition for detoxifying the body insist that the most important factor is eating correctly on a daily basis.

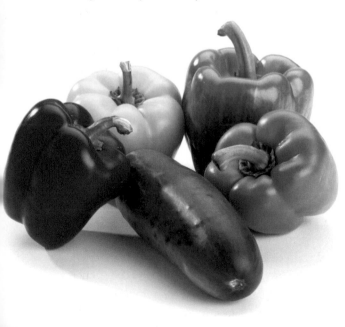

Foods that protect your body

To protect your liver from toxic build-up, you need foods, which we call transformers and escorts; they have shown themselves to be the best places to start when you are expanding your diet.

The transformers

Here's what you can do to help your liver with its first job: transforming toxic substances into intermediate chemicals that can later be removed from your body.

Eat more foods rich in vitamin C These include citrus fruits, red peppers, papaya, cantaloupe, broccoli and tomatoes.

Learn to love limonene This powerful detoxifier is found in citrus fruits such as oranges, lemons, limes and tangerines.

Go easy on grapefruit The one citrus exception is grapefruit. While grapefruit does contain limonene, it also has a substance that actually slows down the first stage of detoxification. If you're taking prescription drugs, for instance, the drugs will clear from your body more slowly if you eat a lot of grapefruit.

Grapefruit also hinders your body's ability to rid itself of the toxic effects of alcohol, which makes mixed drinks that include grapefruit a 'double whammy'. It's fine to eat grapefruit in moderation, but you should probably forgo it altogether if you work in a polluted environment, take a lot of medication or drink too much alcohol.

Get more vitamin E The best food sources are nuts, seeds and vegetable oils. Since it's hard to get all the vitamin E you need from food, you can safely take a daily supplement of 150 International Units (IUs).

Make sure you get enough B vitamins You can increase your B vitamin intake with brewer's yeast, lean beef, chicken, eggs, kidney beans, chickpeas, peanuts, whole wheat flour, brown rice, cheese and other dairy products. If you're a vegetarian, it is possible to get adequate amounts of B vitamins by eating whole grains and dairy products, but do take a B_{12} supplement.

Reach for the bioflavonoids There are hundreds of them, found in a variety of fruits, vegetables and beans. They are also found in tea, which is a really good reason to switch from coffee to tea, at least for some of the time. And if you drink green or black tea, you get the added benefit of the anti-oxidant catechin, which not only protects against heart disease and cancer, but also boosts metabolism. If you prefer caffeine-free tea, remember that removing caffeine also reduces the catechin content.

Boost your brassicas Foods from the brassica family actually help to support both stages of your liver's detoxification efforts. These include cabbage, broccoli, kale and pak choi.

The escorts

Here are some additional suggestions for eating to support the second stage of your liver's detoxification efforts. This phase takes place in several separate steps, turning those intermediate chemicals from stage one into water-soluble substances that can be escorted from your body.

Make lots of glutathione Your body needs good protein to make this important detoxifier. Besides lean meats, you can get protein from dairy products, eggs and beans. It also helps if you eat sulphur-containing foods, such as cabbage, garlic, onions, eggs and red peppers.

Remember molybdenum You're probably not used to thinking about this trace mineral, but your liver loves it. It's found in whole grains and beans.

Learn to love curries Turmeric, a key spice in curries, slows down the first phase of the liver's detoxification efforts, but it speeds up the second phase. That means that when you eat turmeric, you're less likely to have a problem with a build-up of the intermediate toxic chemicals. **Note:** It is possible to buy turmeric in capsules called curcumin and take this detoxifying herb as a supplement.

Gut check

Of course, your liver is not your only detoxifying organ. There's another organ, in which most of your food digestion and absorption actually takes place. It's your small intestine, otherwise known as your gut, and it actually does the digesting.

Your small intestine, which is a thin tube about 6m (20ft) long, is not as small as it seems. This organ is lined by a rough field of microscopic fingers called villi and microvilli. If you flattened it out, it would be the size of a tennis court. It is lined with capillaries, tiny blood vessels that absorb nutrients directly from your small intestine and carry them to your liver and then on to waiting hungry cells throughout your body.

The small intestine is designed to let only the good stuff into your blood and to block out the bad – the toxins from bacteria, from your food, and from any pollutants that ride in on your food. But if you are allergic or even just sensitive to a food, your small intestine can get irritated or even inflamed, and start to leak the contents of your intestine, which include undigested food, thriving colonies of bacteria and waste matter. A lot of it is toxic stuff that you don't want in your bloodstream.

If your intestine starts letting some of it through – this is known as a leaky gut – your immune system views the substance as alien and acts accordingly. If the substance happens to be a partially digested food, your immune system will react to that food the next time it appears.

Sorting out problem foods

If you've ever eaten a food that gives you that 'my stomach is on fire' feeling, you're almost right. What you're feeling is inflammation.

Life would be a lot easier if every food you were sensitive to gave you a 'tummy on fire' reaction. Then those foods would be easy to identify and eliminate. Instead, food sensitivities show up as other kinds of symptom, things like joint pain, fatigue, skin disorders, sinus problems and headaches. It's fairly easy to find out that you're allergic to a food. Food allergies usually cause such dramatic negative reactions that you soon work out that you're allergic. Food sensitivities, on the other hand, are a little harder to pinpoint. In fact, people often crave the very foods that they are sensitive to.

The elimination diet – a special kind of diet that lasts just a few weeks – helps people to find out which foods they are sensitive to.

The most common offenders are dairy products, wheat, chocolate, oranges, corn and soya. All of these are perfectly healthy foods, fine for most people, problematic only for those who are sensitive to them.

There are also foods that are not typical offenders. Some people are sensitive to just one vegetable or fruit, or just tropical fruits. A few people are sensitive to rice, which is supposed to be one of the least likely foods to cause bad reactions.

The elimination diet is the 'gold standard' for finding out which foods you're sensitive to so you can get them out of your diet.

A supervised elimination diet is done right after a brief fast. The idea is to add foods back in one at a time while watching carefully for reactions.

The reactions may be as obvious as a rash or as subtle as the sniffles. Reactions may also include headaches, runny nose, hives, gastrointestinal symptoms such as diarrhoea, wind or abdominal discomfort, or even emotional reactions, such as anxiety or depression. If you discover that you're sensitive to a particular food, your best bet is to either eliminate it entirely or to eat it only on rare occasions, in moderation.

Unfortunately, it's difficult to do an elimination diet on your own. A health care practitioner who is experienced in supervising this procedure begins with taking a thorough medical history that is likely to reveal suspect foods right from the start. As you resume eating after a fast, foods are carefully reintroduced one at a time.

The problem with trying an elimination diet on your own is that it's dangerously easy to either trigger an eating disorder or revive an old eating disorder. And it's easy to make a mistake, either refusing to believe that a favourite food is actually causing a reaction or to misinterpret results and needlessly eliminate a food that's perfectly harmless and is, in fact, really good for you.

Eliminating foods that you are sensitive to can make a dramatic difference in your health. Plugging that leaky gut can bring a level of improvement to such wide-ranging health problems as arthritis symptoms, migraines, chronic fatigue, many skin conditions, obesity and numerous other digestive disorders.

While you need supervision to do an elimination diet, there are a number of things you can do on your own, in addition to eating a nature-based diet from the earth, to promote your body's ongoing detoxification efforts.

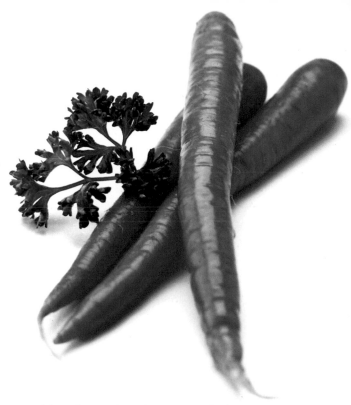

Juice up your life

One of the most efficient ways to take advantage of the multitude of nutrients in fruits and vegetables is through juicing. Juicing simply allows you to take in more nutrients. Your liver loves juices. Your small intestine loves juices. And so do all the other organs in your body.

If you eat a carrot, you get the nutrients of one carrot. Even the most avid health enthusiast is not going to sit and eat eight carrots at one sitting. But you can juice eight carrots with relative ease. They will yield approximately 1 cup of delicious juice that is so full of nutrients that it almost feels electric after it goes down, especially if you drink it while fasting. In fact, many experts who supervise therapeutic fasts recommend supporting your detoxifying efforts with freshly made juices whenever you fast.

Juices are absorbed easily and are also an easy way to get all the nutrients that you need to help your body to do its cleansing and detoxifying work on a daily basis. They support a fast, and they also support your daily diet. When you drink juices throughout the day, your body gets the nutrients it needs to support the detox process.

Although juice bars that prepare fresh juices are proliferating around the country, many towns still don't have even one. And machines that juice vegetables are not exactly cheap. So should you take the plunge?

If you're serious about detoxifying your body, and especially if you plan to fast on a regular basis, the answer is yes. But only if you're going to really use the machine. Just as there are lots of treadmills and exercise bikes sitting unused in dusty corners, there are plenty of juicing machines hidden away in kitchen cabinets.

There are two keys to buying a machine that you will use on a regular basis.

Look for easy cleanup Unless you're going to be juicing for a large family, consider buying a machine that uses a filter. (If you routinely juice for several people at a time, you'll have to change the filter so often that it's impractical.) Then, instead of having to deal with fruit and vegetable fibres that get into every nook and cranny of the machine, you simply pull out the filter and toss it into the compost. You can clean the machine parts afterward with just a quick rinse.

Try new recipes Buy a few books that contain juice recipes and try new ones on a regular basis. If you do, you're more likely to continue using your juicer. The 'I can't believe that tasted so fabulous' recipes will keep you coming back for more.

If you use the juicer often enough in the first months after you buy it, you'll begin to see the difference in your body and feel the difference that it makes in your health. Then you'll be hooked. In any case, if you're going to fast on a regular basis, you need a juicer.

Clean up your food act

We've been talking about making the kinds of food choices that will help your body's efforts to detoxify. But it's also important to clean up your food act, literally.

Choose organic produce whenever possible You can detoxify your body as much as you like, but if you continue to take in more poisons, you're more or less running on the spot. Study after study has shown that pesticide residues are found in non-organic produce. (Some residues are even found in organic produce, but the quantities are minute in comparison.)

While pesticide residues are not good for anybody – especially children and the elderly – some people are more sensitive than others. These are the 'canaries' of our society. (Miners used to take canaries down into the mines to alert them when poison gases were present. When the canary keeled over, the miners would get out of the mine.) The ever-increasing numbers of people with asthma, chronic fatigue, skin conditions, joint pain and cancer are the canaries, letting us all know that we're being exposed to too many pollutants. Short of moving, there's not much you can do about poisons in the air; however, you can limit the poisons you consume by turning to organic produce and by limiting the amount of processed food that you eat.

Learn the secret signs of a clean restaurant Food poisoning comes from toxic bacteria. Just about everyone has experienced an episode of vomiting or diarrhoea after eating in a restaurant, but food poisoning can be bad enough to kill.

Many of the decisions that you make every day can make a significant difference in whether your body's detoxification efforts are being adequately supported. Here's how to add detoxifying foods to your life:

Buy real yogurt Your body contains a lot of bacteria. Amazingly enough, there are more bacteria in your gut than there are cells in your body. You have a pretty important relationship with them, too. When you have the right kind of bacteria in your gut, they help you to digest your food and keep the bad bacteria from moving in.

Whenever you use antibiotics, you kill off the bad bacteria that you're targeting and the good ones, as well. If you fast, many bacteria get flushed away. And as you age, the right kind of bacteria can move out, to be replaced by bad ones.

To keep the right kind of bacterial colonies thriving in your gut, it's helpful to eat yogurt that contains 'live cultures' on a regular basis. Read the label to make sure it specifically says that the micro-organisms are *Lactobacillus acidophilus*. These 'good' bacteria will take up residence in your gut, taking the place of the kind of 'bad' bacteria.

Note It's no longer enough to simply look f or 'live cultures' on the label. Some yogurt manufacturers have found that other kinds of bacteria work better as thickeners, while still delivering a tasty product. But although the bacteria that they are using won't hurt you, they are not able to provide the health-giving functions of *Lactobacillus*.

Fortunately, you can still find good commercial yogurt if you take the trouble to read the label. It's a good idea to buy plain yogurt, not the flavoured kind, and drizzle it with honey or maple syrup, add a handful of berries or chopped peaches and a sprinkle of your favorite nuts.

Buy real juice Of course, it's best to make your own juice. But if you're like most people, you sometimes need the convenience of prepared juices. Don't assume that a juice product that you buy in a natural food store is healthy. Some expensive juices are full of sugar and 'natural flavours' that are only remotely related to fruit juice. Make sure you read the labels.

Expand your garlic repertoire Garlic does a couple of detoxification jobs for you. First, it contains nutrients that help the second phase of your liver's detoxification system. Second, it helps to eliminate harmful bacteria and yeasts from your intestines.

There are numerous ways to enjoy raw garlic. Try adding it to the next commercial frozen pizza that you heat up. (We're assuming here that you're not eating things like commercial frozen pizza every night!)

Follow the package directions for cooking it, but then slide the pizza out exactly a minute before it's done. Sprinkle a tablespoon (or two, if you can take it) of finely chopped garlic on top of the pizza. Then put it back into the oven and let it cook for one more minute.

A handful of raw garlic is also great on pasta drizzled with a little olive oil and sprinkled with grated Parmesan cheese.

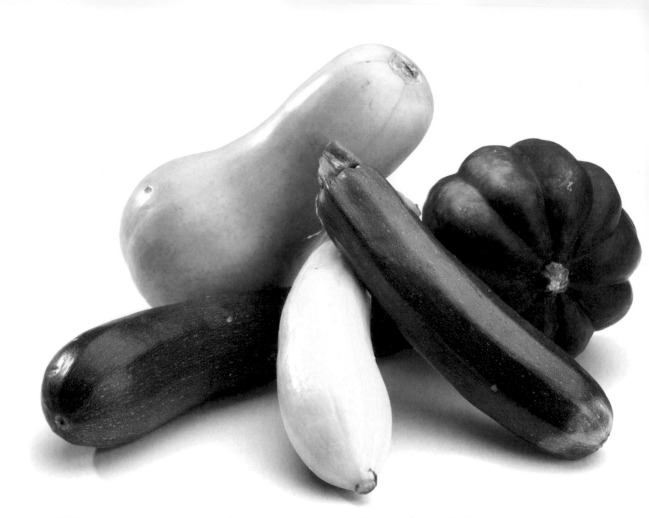

While there's never a way to be 100 percent certain that a restaurant's kitchen is clean, here's a tip from the long-time owner of an Italian restaurant. Look at three things in a restaurant:

- The restroom area
- The menus
- Any glass around the entrance

If the owner of the restaurant doesn't take steps to see that these things that are seen by the public are kept clean, there's a good chance that the kitchen is filthy. Find somewhere else to eat.

Strictly avoid anything that's rancid Nuts that taste a little odd? Cooking oil with a slightly 'off' smell? You might be tempted to nibble the nuts or use the oil anyway – but don't!

Avoid restaurants that smell of hot, rancid oil, too. Rancid oils won't make you obviously sick the way spoiled meat can. But rancid oils produce vast numbers of free radicals – very active oxygen molecules that do serious damage in the body. Bad oils are seriously toxic, contribute to ageing and can even trigger cancerous changes in cells.

Set realistic limits If fruits and vegetables are good for you, what about going on a diet that's exclusively fruits and vegetables? What about being a vegetarian or vegan? What about the raw foods diet that's getting so much attention of late? What about macrobiotics?

Any diet that incorporates a lot of fruits and vegetables is good for you. And it's good for you precisely because it contains lots of fruits and vegetables as well as other foods. Vegetarianism and veganism can be healthy diets, but adherents need to be careful that they don't end up with chronic deficiencies in proteins, essential fatty acids and minerals.

TAKE A PASS ON PURGATIVES

There's much hype about using powerful laxatives as super-detox agents.

Herbs like aloe, dock, and senna will make you rush to the toilet feeling like a bullet train is about to arrive. The immediate results are impressive, but the problem with these herbs is that you end up losing more than toxins. You can also lose important minerals from your body – and you can end up laxative dependent.

Indeed, if you know anything about the history of these herbs, you know that they have no place in a 21st-century detox plan. More than 100 years ago, doctors used treatments like bleeding, mercury, lead and strong herbal laxatives. As bizarre as this may sound, people believed in these. They were given laxatives to the point of death, with the aim of returning them to health. Now we find people using these potentially dangerous herbs in detox regimens. The best advice is to avoid powerful laxatives altogether.

Water fit to drink

Today, in many places, people use some kind of filter or purifier to treat drinking water. Whether you should or not may depend on where you live. Although water standards in Europe are generally high, they do vary from place to place.

To determine whether you need to treat the water you drink, first find out what, if any, unhealthy contaminants are lurking in it.

Get the report Contact your local water supply company about the cleanliness of the water it supplies. Ask if you can have a water quality report. Also, ask if the company has found high levels of any of the contaminants it tests for voluntarily and what steps have been taken to remove the contaminants.

Read the fine print Go into detail about the contents of the water. It may get an overall safe rating but be high in certain contaminants.

If you are pregnant or have an infant at home, look for levels of nitrate, a contaminant from fertilizer and faeces, and chlorination by-products called trihalomethanes. These may increase risks of miscarriage, birth defects and other health problems. Facts may be buried in the fine print.

If your children are six years old or younger, it may be a good idea to test for lead, even if your water supplier's report shows low levels of this toxic metal in your water supply. These days, lead contamination may originate inside the house.

Most cities have replaced old lead water mains, but older buildings may may still have lead pipes or copper pipes welded with leaded solder.

Find the right treatment

If you do find something in your water, which treatment system should you use? Again, that depends on what's in there, on whether you want to treat every drop that enters your home and on how much you're willing to spend. There are several different types of treatment devices, from carbon filters to more complex ion exchange systems and distillers.

Unfortunately, there's no single system that removes all contaminants. So you might need more than one device. Most types come in a variety of models. Trawl the internet for full details of all the water filtering systems available. Weigh up the pros and cons against your needs.

Chapter 4
The essential herbs
Nature's best purifiers

When people talk about detox programmes, the subject of herbal medicines always comes up. And it's true: herbs do have a role in a detoxification programme. Here's how to incorporate them into your lifestyle in a way that suits you.

Although you may have heard about using herbs for detox purposes, you may not know where or how to begin. What herb should you use? For how long should you use it? What dose should you take? As soon as you move from talking about using herbs for detox to actually taking them, things start to get tricky.

This chapter includes the most important information you need about using herbs for purification. It will help you to find the best detox herbs to meet your personal needs and create a sensible herbal detox programme that will really make a difference in your life.

Ancient herbal healing secrets

For centuries, human beings have used herbs for this purpose. The toxins may have changed, but using herbs to get toxins out of the body before they make you sick has been an accepted practice since the beginning of written history.

Whereas most mushrooms are harmless, some deliver a toxic punch that destroys the liver along with the person who owns it. Long ago, mushroom gatherers learned that if you accidentally ate a bad mushroom, milk thistle (*Silybum marianum*) could help you to survive.

The 15th century Italian noblewoman Lucretia Borgia and other European nobles resolved more than one disagreement with the aid of poison – for some rulers, poisoning people who got in your way was standard procedure. The food tasters employed by the European nobility were not mere status symbols. They risked their lives, one taste at a time, to keep a ruler safe from malicious poisoning. If a taster was poisoned, Mithradites treacle was used to counteract the effects of the poison. Concocted from herbs, this antidote was used to detoxify the body and ensure survival. Success rates are not recorded.

Poisoning was not just a political affair. John Gerard, a famous 16th-century English herbalist, tells us that it was also a domestic problem. Gerard cautioned stepchildren to keep a supply of lemons around the house to counteract the poisoning they might expect from their stepmothers. According to Gerard, lemons worked against the diverse poisons at the disposal of the most determined 'wicked stepmothers' of the day.

In North America, Native Americans knew all about toxins. The tribes dealt with two sorts. The first were toxins injected into the body by poisonous creatures, such as rattlesnakes and scorpions. The second were toxins delivered by the tip of an arrow. In both cases, the Native Americans used echinacea to detoxify the poisons injected into the body by beast or enemy.

Globally, herbs were also used to detoxify toxins of a less sinister nature: toxins produced by the body itself. Long winters, short on green vegetables and rich in meat and potatoes, meant people felt pretty bad by springtime. The traditional solution to this seasonal problem was a spring tonic. In Europe, people gathered spring greens, dandelion, watercress and chicory to help the body to rid itself of stored toxins. In North America, they brewed white pine needles, Douglas fir fronds and sassafras bark into spring-cleaning teas.

Researchers have spent years scrutinizing these long-used remedies. In the process, they have discovered the hidden secrets of these herbs. Many of the old remedies' uses have been validated through scientific scrutiny. In some cases, study has even highlighted new uses for these herbs. Empowered by this knowledge, we have the opportunity to use herbal detox agents with unprecedented precision and accuracy.

KEYS TO SUCCESS WITH HOUSEKEEPING HERBS

Housekeeping herbs can be used to boost your body's natural capacity to rid itself of toxins by helping to stimulate urination, sweating and defecation. Here are some tips for using them properly.

• Select one herb that strengthens your weakness. If you don't urinate a lot, use a diuretic herb to increase urination. If you don't sweat much, use an herb that increases sweating. If you are prone to constipation, choose one with laxative qualities, and so on.

• Stick with one herb. Plan to use that herb for a solid month. This will go a long way towards getting toxins out of your system.

• After a month of using a housekeeping herb, discontinue its use, but don't forget about it completely. Detox is not a once-a-year proposition. It's something we need to attend to all the time. So bring back the herb for a full week every month to maintain your detoxification and keep your whole system clean.

Your herbal detox strategies

Scientists have divided the miracle plants into two basic categories:

- Herbs that increase the body's excretion of toxins (housekeeping herbs).
- Herbs that increase the body's resistance to toxins (resistance herbs).

To use herbs most effectively for safe yet powerful purification, our simple, three-step approach combines herbs from both of these categories and adds an anti-toxin beverage.

- Select a 'housekeeping' herb and use it for one month.
- Select a 'resistance-raising' herb and use it periodically, when you need special protection.
- Add an anti-toxin beverage to your shopping list and use it regularly.

Here are your options for each of these steps. You'll discover the herbs you should consider for your personal purification plan.

Note Talk to your health care practitioner before adding herbal remedies to your diet.

1 Select a housekeeping herb

Practitioners of herbal medicine believe in working with the body and never against it. They use certain herbs to encourage the body to do what it does naturally. This is where the housekeeping herbs come in – they are taken to stimulate the toxin removal system.

You already know about certain foods that have this capacity. You have probably eaten too many prunes and found yourself spending a few extra minutes on the toilet the next day. Or perhaps you've had a big cup of coffee before hitting the road and ended up desperately looking for the nearest rest stop. Ever eat a hot pepper and break out in big beads of sweat? These are all examples of herbs and foods stimulating the organs of toxin removal into dynamic action. There are lots of herbs that get these systems going.

Though you probably know that your digestive tract, urinary tract, and skin move toxins out of your body, you may not know that your immune system has a role to play. The immune cells patrol the body looking for bacteria, viruses and cancer, and when they spot trouble, they collect it and dispose of it. The immune cells also pick up toxins. They search the cracks and crevices of your body for toxic substances, and if they spot any, they sweep them up. The immune system is the silent star of our natural detox ability.

Herbal medicines can be used to increase your body's efficiency. There are a number of herbal immune system stimulants that increase the number of immune cells produced by the body and the activity of the existing immune cells. They get the immune cells working.

The best herb to do this job is the herb that matches your weakness with strength. Identify your personal weakness, and then select a herb that counters this weakness. (See 'Keys to success with housekeeping herbs' on page 35.) Choose from these excellent housekeeping options.

Buchu The kidney stimulant

Scientific name *Barosma betulina*
Part used Leaf
Best for:
Urinary tract infections Contains compounds that kill the bacteria that cause urinary tract infections and other compounds that soothe irritated urinary tissues.
Kidney stones Holding urine for too long gives stones the chance to form. This herb gets the urine flowing so that stones can't form.
Infrequent urination Regular urination means toxins are constantly whisked out of your body. Buchu contains oils that increase urine production.

What it does Buchu is an aromatic herb rich in volatile oils that give the spicy leaves their fruity, blackcurrant taste. These oils stimulate the kidney cells to increase activity. The leaves also contain mucilage, resins and tannins thought to contribute to the diuretic effect. Non-toxic buchu is so safe it is used in popular herbal teas.

Using buchu The best way to use good-tasting buchu is in the form of a hot tea. Buy buchu leaves at the health food shop. Boil water and add 1 teaspoon of leaves to 1 cup of water. Let them infuse for 5 minutes, strain, and drink while still hot. Three cups of this tea per day is the recommended dosage. For major detoxification, think about using buchu every day for a month. After this, use buchu several times a month to keep toxins flowing where you want them to flow – down the drain.

Origins Buchu is an aromatic shrub native to South Africa. When the European colonists first arrived, they encountered buchu. Long used by the Hottentot tribe as a cleansing herb and vitality tonic, it was not long before buchu was traded internationally. It was shipped from Africa to London, and then on to North America to be used as a urinary stimulant. At the beginning of the 19th century, it had become one of America's most popular urinary tonics.

Detox! dosage

Take One dose, three times a day
One dose = 1 cup of buchu leaf tea
(see above for instructions)
or 1 teaspoon of tincture 1:5
or 20 drops of tincture 1:1

Dandelion Liver stimulant

Scientific name *Taraxacum officinalis*
Part used Root
Best for:
Sluggish digestion Increases digestive gland activity. This causes speedy digestion, absorption and then excretion of waste.
Constipation Increases bile production. Bile has a natural laxative effect, so constipation improves and waste excretion is increased.
Mild liver insufficiency Activates blood-cleansing liver cells. If your liver is performing poorly, dandelion can be used to give it gentle encouragement.

What it does The root contains a collection of compounds that stimulate waste removal on several levels, in the liver, the kidneys and the immune system.

Dandelion is a mild laxative. However, its laxative effect is rooted in its detoxifying action. As the liver cleanses the blood, it deposits the waste products into bile. The liver then ships the bile into the gallbladder and the gallbladder in turn ships the bile into the intestine. Out go the toxins. Bile has many physiological actions, including a laxative effect. When you take dandelion you get increased liver cleansing and a reduction in constipation.

Using dandelion Many a case of chronic constipation has been eased with its use.

Dandelion root is available at health food shops. Add 1 teaspoon of the root to 2 cups of boiling water. Boil the root for 15 minutes to extract all of its medicinal attributes. Take 1 cup three times a day. It is probably easiest to make the whole day's tea in the morning. You can reheat the tea in a saucepan or in the microwave as the day goes along. For a major detox, think about using dandelion tea every day for a month. After that, use it occasionally to keep your system free of toxins. You may find it easier to take a tincture rather than make the tea.

However, don't try to use the plant from your garden – pesticides, fertilizers and the habits of roaming cats and dogs mean it is not worth the risk. Besides, the herb is quite inexpensive to buy.

Detox! dosage

Take One dose, three times a day.

One dose = 1 cup of dandelion root tea (see above for instructions)

or Two 500mg tablets of tableted dandelion root

or 1 teaspoon of tincture 1:5

or 20 drops of tincture 1:1

Origins Dandelion has spread itself around the globe. In Europe, Asia, Africa and South America, dandelion has long been used to rid the body of unhealthy toxins. For thousands of years, people have used it in spring detox regimens and when retention of toxins has caused illness.

Echinacea Immune system stimulant

Scientific name *Echinacea purpurea*
Part used Root
Best for:

Recurrent urinary, skin, or respiratory infections Stimulates the production and activity of white blood cells responsible for keeping infection under control. Echinacea can be used to relieve chronic infections.

Possible cancer prevention Activates the immune system. People susceptible to cancer need to know about this herb. The immune system is responsible for destroying cancer cells before they have the chance to take hold.

Exposure to infectious disease Stimulates the immune system.

Warning Echinacea must not be used by people with auto-immune diseases such as muscular dystrophy (MS).

What it does Echinacea stimulates both the production and activity of immune cells. When you use echinacea, there are more immune cells combing the body for toxins, and they are doing it at an accelerated rate.

Using echinacea If your immune system is letting bacteria and viruses survive, it's also likely to be leaving toxins in place. To increase your immune function, use echinacea.

When you buy an echinacea product, look for a product made of the root of *Echinacea purpurea*. Many companies are marketing products made from leaves and flowers, and you want to avoid those. Though you can make a tea out of loose dried root (just boil 1 teaspoon of dried root in 1 cup of water for 10 minutes), it's easier to use tablets. For a big cleanse, think about using echinacea for a month. After that, use echinacea occasionally to keep your body free of toxins.

Detox! dosage

Take One dose, three times a day.

One dose = 1 cup of loose dry root tea (see below left for instructions)

or One 500mg tablet of tableted echinacea root

or 1 teaspoon of tincture 1:5

or 20 drops of tincture 1:1

Origins Echinacea was first used by the Native Americans to treat rattlesnake, scorpion and tarantula bites. When a venomous insect or animal bites, they inject venom into the body. The immune system sends in immune cells to vacuum the toxins out before they can do any damage. Native Americans found that echinacea prevented the gangrene caused by snake-bites. It expelled the snake venom before the poison could destroy the tissues surrounding the bite.

Elder Skin stimulant

Scientific name *Sambucus nigra*
Part used Flower
Best for:
Lack of sweating Opens up the sweat glands and gets them pumping toxins out of the body.
Poor circulation Gently increases circulation. It causes a warm glow shortly after a person drinks a hot cup of the tea.
Coughs and colds Can be used to break a fever. More importantly, it stimulates the immune system to nip a cold in the bud or shorten the duration of a cold.
Warning Pregnant women should avoid it as it has a laxative effect.

What it does It contains chemicals that increase circulation to the sweat glands. With blood nourishing the glands, the glands produce sweat.
Using elder This is another easy-to-use remedy. Put 1 teaspoon of the flowers in 1 cup of boiling water, allow it to infuse for 5 minutes, then strain, and it will work its magic. If you want to increase its detox effect, add a teaspoon of honey and lemon juice to your cup of hot tea. For a proper cleanout, think about using elder three times a day for a month. After that, use it for an occasional cleanup.

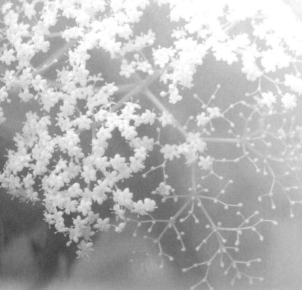

Detox! dosage

Take One dose, three times a day.
One dose = 1 cup of elder flower tea
(see above for instructions)
or 1 teaspoon of tincture 1:5
or 20 drops of tincture 1:1

Origins The elder tree is a European native long used for a wide variety of purposes. The stems and leaves are made into healing salves, and the berries are made into vitality-stimulating syrups. The flowers are used as a remedy for coughs, colds, fevers and water retention. Officially speaking, the flowers are termed diaphoretic, meaning they increase the sweat glands' production of sweat. Historically, elder's ability to increase sweating is the reason it was used to break a fever.

2 Select a resistance herb

Resistance herbs, also known as adaptogens, are herbal medicines that raise resistance to toxins. Researchers have shown that adaptogens make the body less susceptible to toxin damage. In the toxin-laden world we live in, we all need increased resistance to toxins. To take full advantage of this type of herbal medicine, you need some background information.

Everyone knows that exhaust from cars, lead, preservatives, artificial colours, flavours and sweeteners, and the like, are bad for our health.

Beginning in the 1940s, researchers began studying stress. Specifically, a Canadian researcher named Hans Selye took an interest in the subject. Selye found that when a person is exposed to a toxic substance, regardless of the nature of the toxin, a generalized physical reaction occurs. Initially, the body responds with shock. Then the body adapts to the toxin. Selye found that over time, this adaptation fails. The body can resist the toxin for only so long. Once resistance fails, all kinds of physiological abnormalities set in. Selye noticed hormone abnormalities (both overproduction and underproduction), immune abnormalities (such as allergies, psoriasis, eczema, arthritis, asthma and ulcerative colitis) and nervous abnormalities (including depression, anxiety and learning deficits). And these are just a few of the problems that can develop.

The original stress scientist, Selye felt that the solution was to find substances that increased resistance to toxic compounds. A Russian researcher, Israel Brekhman, was fascinated with the work of Selye and set out to find substances that raised the body's resistance to all forms of stress, and to toxic compounds in particular. He found these substances and called them adaptogens because they help the body adapt to resisting toxins.

When we talk about herbal medicine and detoxification, the adaptogen is of primary importance. Our bodies are bombarded by toxins daily. Adaptogens increase our bodies' ability to withstand them.

Since the start of adaptogen research in the 1950s, a lot has been learned. At present, we have a host of adaptogens available to us. You need to find the adaptogen that most suits your particular circumstances. Although all adaptogens raise resistance to toxins, each one has a particular strength. Here are some to choose from:

Ashwagandha A tonic

Scientific name *Withania somnifera*
Part used Root
Best for:
The elderly Used to strengthen the elderly and decrease symptoms of ageing.
The ill Increases the vitality and resistance of those suffering from chronic disease.
The stressed It raises resistance in those who have been afflicted by stress or serious health problems.

What it does Researchers have demonstrated that ashwagandha increases resistance to many forms of stress, limiting the damaging effects of stress on the nerves. The herb acts as a powerful anti-oxidant, neutralizing some of the internal toxins produced by the body itself.

Using Ashwagandha This is a traditional tonic for all who are less able to resist toxins. It can be used long-term.

Detox! dosage

Take One dose, twice a day.

One dose = 1½ teaspoons of dried root powder, taken morning and night.
(Traditionally this is added to boiling milk, though it can be taken simply as a powder mixed with some boiling water.)

or Two 250mg tablets of standardized extract

Origins Ashwagandha is native to India, where it is a major component in traditional ayurvedic medicine; it is viewed as a tonic and aphrodisiac, and is used to strengthen the vulnerable against the stresses of life. It is said to make the weak strong and the strong stronger. If you are in any way compromised in your ability to resist stress and disease, think about using ashwagandha.

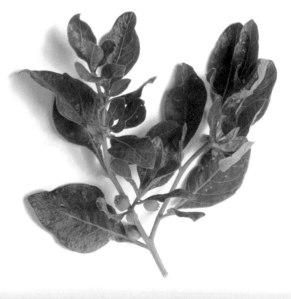

Siberian ginseng All-purpose resistance booster

Scientific name *Eleutherococcus senticosus*
Part used Root
Best for:
Working mothers Reduces the damage done to the body by a demanding schedule.
Cancer treatment support Used to raise resistance to the side effects of cancer therapies and to speed recovery from them. Research indicates it also has a role in preventive regimens.
Athletes Long used by professional athletes to help their bodies to recover from the stress of arduous exercise. Numerous studies have established that it increases stamina and reduces wear and tear.
Warning Do not use if you have high blood pressure.

What it does Research reveals that Siberian ginseng raises resistance to some specific forms of toxic stress, radiation and narcotics. It has also been widely studied in humans. It has, in fact, been administered to more than 2,100 people in 44 separate studies. In these studies, the herb increased individuals' ability to withstand stressors such as toxic compounds.

Siberian ginseng may also be the best herbal medicine for people who are exposed to cancer-causing compounds. Early on, researchers found that it reduced tumours and cancers that had been caused by a variety of chemicals.

Oddly, toxic chemicals cause cancer, and yet are also used to treat cancer. In scientific studies, Siberian ginseng has been shown to protect against radiation and toxic chemotherapy regimens.
Using Siberian ginseng Siberian ginseng is a good all-purpose adaptogen. It's an excellent option for raising your resistance to toxins. It's useful both for those who are occasionally exposed to toxic compounds and for those who are regularly exposed.

KEYS TO SUCCESS WITH RESISTANCE HERBS

Though your body has a built-in ability to resist toxins, it can do so for only so long. At some point, resistance fails and all kinds of health problems set in. That's when resistance herbs, also called adaptogens, can be used to raise resistance to toxins. Here's how:

• Select an adaptogen that is most appropriate to your particular health needs. (Though adaptogens have similar features, they also have individual strengths.)

• Use adaptogens when you are heading into a toxin-rich time, such as when you are going to paint your house, take a flight or go on holiday where it's likely that you'll overindulge.

• Use adaptogens to raise your resistance to toxin exposure if you are routinely exposed to toxic substances. Farm workers, professional gardeners, dry cleaners, hairdressers, chemical factory workers, petrochemical refinery workers, commercial cleaners and hotel staff can all benefit from using adaptogens.

• Use adaptogens to raise your resistance to the toxicity of prescription medications. Over-the-counter and prescription medications, while helpful, also put stress on your body. These compounds were not meant to be in your body, and so your body has to work to get them out. If you regularly take medicine, consider using an adaptogen.

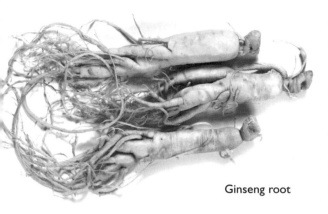

Ginseng root

Ginseng For drinkers, smokers and drug users

Scientific name *Panax ginseng*
Part used Root
Best for:
Smokers Reduces the toxic effects of cigarette smoking and may reduce the risk of cancer.
Drinkers Reduces the toxicity of alcohol and reduces the damage done by drinking. Ginseng can even be used to prevent or reduce hangovers.
Drug takers Increases resistance to toxic drugs. It may have a role in diminishing damage done by both street drugs and prescription drugs.
People addicted to a variety of substances Your body has to spend a lot of time getting really toxic compounds out of your system when it should be attending to other matters. Under these conditions, your body is stressed and needs something to help it out. History and science both reveal that ginseng may offer the necessary boost.
Warning Do not use ginseng if you have high blood pressure.

If you are painting the house, refinishing the floors or treating the grass, use Siberian ginseng for a week following your exposure. If you work with chemicals, and exposure occurs daily, use the herb for one month in every three. If you are going to be exposed to toxins either occasionally or routinely, use the herb to raise your resistance. This is especially important if there is cancer in your family or if it seems to be a particular hazard of your profession.

To make Siberian ginseng tea, add ½ teaspoon of dried root to 1 cup of water and let it boil for 15 minutes. Strain, then drink.

What it does Ginseng has been shown to increase resistance to radiation, toxic chemicals (carbon tetrachloride and thioacetamide) and narcotic and alcohol intoxication.

Among other things, chronic exposure to toxic compounds can cause cancer. Smokers develop lung cancer; drinkers develop liver cancer.

Ginseng increases resistance to cancer. It has been found to inhibit the production of tumours caused by toxins, to inhibit the spread of tumours, to increase tolerance of toxic anti-tumour drugs, and to stimulate the body's natural killer cell activity. Natural killer cells are a part of the immune system that help to eliminate cancer cells from the body. One study also demonstrated that ginseng inhibited the cancer development associated with chronic hepatitis and cirrhosis of the liver.

Detox! dosage

Take One dose, twice a day.

One dose = I cup of dried Siberian ginseng root tea (see left for instructions)

or Two 500mg tablets of dried root

or One I00mg tablet of standardized extract containing I percent or more Siberian ginsengside

or I teaspoon of tincture I:5

or 20 drops of tincture I:I

Origins Siberian ginseng is a thorny shrub found growing in far eastern Russia, north-eastern China, Korea and Japan. Throughout Asia, the herb is used to stimulate vitality and to increase a person's ability to withstand the daily grind.

Using ginseng Ginseng should be used to reduce the damage that regular exposure to toxins does to the body. In other words, if you are regularly putting chemicals into your body, use ginseng regularly but not continuously (one month in three is advised). If you are occasionally putting chemicals into your body, use ginseng occasionally. If exposure is constant, think about using ginseng two weeks out of every month. If exposure is incidental, use ginseng for a week following the exposure.

You can take ginseng in the form of a tea. Just boil 1 teaspoon of dried root in 1 cup of water for 10 to 20 minutes. Strain, then drink.

Detox! dosage

Take One dose daily.

One dose = 1 cup of dried ginseng root tea (see above for instructions)

or Two 500mg tablets of dried root

or One tablet of standardized extract containing 5mg of ginsenosides

or 1 teaspoon root tincture 1:5

or 20 drops root tincture 1:1

Origins In Asia, ginseng has been used for centuries to stimulate the return of health and vitality among the ill and the elderly. Whenever health was challenged by a potentially lethal event, significant injury or poisoning, people reached for ginseng to increase their resistance. Its reputation was so great that herb researchers started examining this plant early on – between 1969 and 2003, more than 2,300 studies were conducted on it. The conclusion is that ginseng really does increase strength and vitality, even when there is something like disease or chronic exposure to toxins undermining well-being.

Milk thistle Counteracts chemicals

Scientific name *Silybum marianum*
Part used Seed
Best for:
Farmers and professional gardeners Agricultural pesticides, herbicides and fertilizers tax the liver and can damage your body. Milk thistle, with its proven ability to protect the liver, can be used to reduce this damage.
Painters, plumbers and electricians Tradesmen are exposed to solvents, lead and a collection of toxic chemicals. Milk thistle can be used to speed the removal of these compounds and protect the liver from damage.
Professional drivers, dry cleaners and photo shop workers These people inhale toxic fumes that are absorbed through the lungs and removed by the liver. Milk thistle can be used to protect the liver from the damaging effects of these toxins.

What it does In 1900, not that many people worked with chemicals, but by 2005, not many people can avoid working with chemicals in some form or another. Naturally, people are concerned about the effects on their health of regular exposure to toxins.

Medically speaking, the liver is largely responsible for getting these compounds out of your system. Milk thistle might be just what you need because research reveals that milk thistle contains flavolignans that protect the liver from damage due to toxic substances. Milk thistle seed contains 3 percent silymarin, which is actually a generic name for the flavolignan compounds that protect the liver. The most active substance is something known as silybin.

Silymarin makes the liver cells less susceptible to damage by toxins. The toxins enter the liver via the blood, but they are not able to do as much damage because milk thistle increases the liver's production of an anti-toxin chemical called glutathione, raising it to 35 percent above normal.

Using milk thistle Milk thistle protects your liver from all sorts of chemical damage, and can be used as a daily tonic. Make a tea by boiling 1 teaspoon of milk thistle seed in 1 cup of water for 10 minutes. Just strain the seed out and drink.

Detox! dosage

Take One dose, three times a day.

One dose = 1 cup of milk thistle seed tea (see above for instructions)

or 2 tablets of standardized extract containing 100mg silymarin, going as high as 600mg per day

or 1 teaspoon milk thistle tincture 1:5

or 20 drops milk thistle tincture 1:1

Origins Native to the Mediterranean, milk thistle has been used since antiquity to protect the liver against damaging diseases and compounds. Arabian physicians working in the 9th century were quite aware of liver disease. Hepatitis was a common condition due to sanitation problems. Milk thistle was widely used then and, later, in European history, it was also used to help people to survive accidental or intentional poisoning. Milk thistle is also known as wild artichoke.

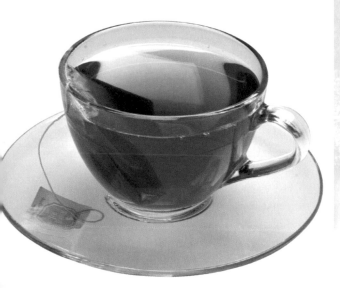

TEA VERSUS TINCTURE

For detox or any other purpose, the key to success is using your selected herbs regularly. As such, the best way to take herbs is the manner in which you are most likely to keep on using them. If you enjoy making and drinking tea, then plan to use herbal teas. If you live life on the run, then tinctures may be a more viable option. Tinctures are easy to transport in a handbag or briefcase. Be realistic and make a plan that you can actually live with.

Using teas The herbs described in this chapter can be purchased in natural food shops, health food shops and, with increasing frequency, in chemists and supermarkets. They're usually available both loose and in tea bags. Which you use is simply a matter of personal preference.

Using tinctures Tinctures are water/alcohol extracts of herbs. A mixture of alcohol and water is passed over the herbs and the herbs' healing principles are captured in the liquid. Importantly, any well-made tincture will have a ratio on the bottle. It will say Tincture 1:4, Tincture 1:3, or something similar. These ratios indicate the strength of the tincture. These numbers are important.

A 1:1 tincture is 10 times as strong as a 1:10 tincture! If you have been directed to take a 1:10 tincture, take a 1:10 tincture; do not assume that more is better. You should not take tinctures straight from the bottle but mix them with tea, juice or water.

Schisandra The liver's protector

Scientific name *Schisandra sinensis*
Part used Berry
Best for:

Drinkers Protects your liver from chronic exposure to toxic substances, including alcohol. If used regularly, it may prevent liver damage.

Chemical workers Speeds the process of removing toxic chemicals from your body and protects your liver from damage. Working with chemicals means your liver has to work double time to get chemicals out of your body.

Poor liver function Improves liver function and thereby speeds toxin removal. When the liver functions below par, toxins remain in your system longer than they should.

What it does Schisandra acts as a free-radical scavenger. It contains nine different compounds that neutralize these damaging substances.

When it comes to its anti-toxic effect, this herb has a remarkable record. In one study, it reduced liver damage associated with an Alzheimer's drug and the very liver-damaging compound carbon tetrachloride.

In study after study, both on animals and humans, schisandra reduced the amount of damage done to the body and, in particular, the liver, when toxic compounds were an issue. And, as with all adaptogens, researchers found that this herb increased general resistance and energy levels while doing its magic.

Using schisandra Beyond its general anti-toxin effects, this herb has some fairly specific uses. First, schisandra has a role in reducing the toxicity associated with drug therapies. In the study that demonstrated schisandra's ability to protect the liver from toxicity associated with one Alzheimer's medication, the efficacy of the drug was not affected. If prescription medicines you need to take are also causing liver damage, think about using schisandra.

Second, the herb has a role in raising liver resistance to toxic compound exposure in workers. Anyone exposed to toxic compounds, either routinely or incidentally, should think about using this herb.

Lastly, schisandra's ability to protect against liver damage suggests that it's a must for those who have a problem with alcohol. Excessive alcohol intake is notoriously damaging to the liver. Once the liver has been damaged, it can't get toxins out of the body efficiently. If alcohol is an issue, schisandra may be the best adaptogen available.

You can take schisandra by drinking a beverage made from the berries. Boil 1½ teaspoons of berries in 1 cup of water for 5 minutes. Strain and drink each morning.

Detox! dosage

Take One dose daily.
One dose = 1 cup of schisandra berry tea

Origins Native to China, schisandra has been used as a tonic for thousands of years and is one of the fundamental herbs in traditional Chinese medicine. Many parts of the plant are used medicinally. For detoxification purposes, the berry is of the greatest interest. Traditionally, it is considered to be an astringent, aphrodisiac, stimulant and tonic. It has been used primarily for night sweats but also for amnesia, asthma, coughs, diabetes, diarrhoea, dysentery, insomnia, premature ejaculation and tuberculosis. Though this seems like a diverse list of conditions, there is a central theme here: the herb raises resistance to whatever is taxing the body.

KEYS TO SUCCESS WITH A HERBAL DETOX

Here's how to make herbs your most trusted allies in your detoxification efforts.

• Create a detox regimen that you can maintain. Think long term and try to avoid Herculean efforts. It's better to add one herb to your regular programme and stick with it than to go overboard and quit in a few weeks.

• Think ahead. If you know you are going to paint the house, fertilize the lawn, overindulge or in some way be exposed to toxins, use a resistance herb to raise your resistance to chemicals. When the exposure is over, use a housekeeping herb to speed the removal of toxins.

• Know that your body has the capacity to deal with toxins. Your liver, kidneys, sweat glands and immune system are all in place to get toxins out of your body. Work with your body, using herbal medicine to increase this capacity.

• Choose to drink an anti-toxin instead of a beverage that contains toxins. Making this simple change will make an enormous difference in your health.

• Make herbal detox a regular part of your life. Like exercise, it's something you should think about every day.

3 Add an anti-toxin drink

Whatever people drink, they tend to drink routinely. If you drink toxin-laden beverages (those containing caffeine or alcohol) all the time, you are constantly flooding your body with toxins. Alternatively, if you drink anti-toxin beverages regularly, you fill your body with toxin-neutralizing refreshment. Getting into the habit of drinking good-for-you beverages goes a long way toward taking care of the toxin problem.

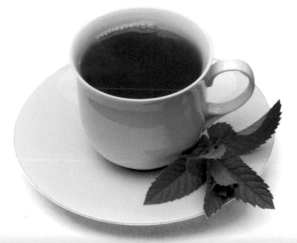

ANTI-TOXIN BEVERAGES

There is a wide range of anti-toxins coming from the plant kingdom. If you can find red sorrel tea, it is considered the best, but you can also get really great detox benefits from adding these refreshing drinks to your diet:

• Apple juice
• Cranberry juice
• Douglas fir frond tea
• Grape juice
• Green tea
• White pine needle tea

Chapter 5

Get moving
Building a better, cleaner body

Imagine yourself as a body of water. Given the choice, would you rather be a stagnant pond, collecting debris, pollution and bacteria, or a mountain stream, splashing through rocks and flora, filtering out dirt and impurities?

Although the analogy may be a bit of an oversimplification, your body works much like these two waters. It collects disease-causing toxins when you're sedentary, and it runs itself clean when you move.

In addition to all the toxins in the environment, that affect us, we also make our own 'toxins' in the form of cellular waste and excess hormones such as oestrogen. Left unchecked, all toxins can poison the body.

Some signs of accumulating inner 'gunk' are everyday problems like fatigue, sluggishness, headaches, digestive problems and assorted skin conditions. But toxins that the body does not throw off may even be implicated in long-term chronic diseases such as heart disease or arthritis.

Purification in motion

Experts have only recently begun linking the detoxifying power of exercise with important health benefits.

Just as there's more than one way that toxins infiltrate your system, there's more than one way that exercise helps to flush them out. The following are the most well-documented ways in which physical exercise helps you to detoxify.

The purification patrol
A healthy lymphatic system is key to keeping your immune system in top working condition. Disease-fighting white blood cells are stored in your lymph nodes, a major group of lymph vessels

THE POTENTIAL CANCER-OBESITY CONNECTION

Some research suggests that being overweight increases your risk for cancers of various kinds. The Mayo Clinic compared women of a healthy weight with obese women and found that obese women may have:

- Up to 1½ times greater risk for breast cancer after menopause
- 2 to 4 times the risk of endometrial cancer
- 2 to 4 times the risk of kidney cancer
- 2 times the risk of pancreatic cancer
- 46 percent higher risk of developing colon cancer

which are located under your arms, at your neck and around your spine and groin. These cells are carried by lymphatic fluid throughout your body.

A study on immunity likens immune cells to policemen. When you're sedentary, they sit about in the station, or lymph tissue, where they are fairly inactive. Almost as soon as you start exercising, however, and for a few hours afterwards, they pull out of the station and patrol your body, seeking out and destroying invading bacteria and viruses. In one study, when 150 people walked regularly for twelve weeks, they had about half the number of sore throats and colds as their sedentary peers.

Lymph also does double-duty as a rubbish collector. While sweeping through your system, lymph fluid filters out and carries away cellular waste and other toxins, so they can be processed and removed from your body.

There is two to three times as much lymphatic fluid in your body as blood. Yet unlike blood, which is pushed through your body at the amazing rate of 6 litres (10½ pints) a minute by your heart, your lymphatic system moves very little until you do, relying mostly on muscle compression on the lymphatic vessels to keep the fluid circulating.

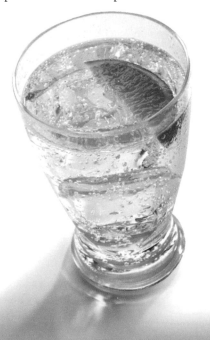

So the best way to keep it flowing is to exercise every day. Regular physical activity not only keeps the lymph circulating on a regular basis, it also improves your general range of flexibility and motion, and your body posture – all of which help to keep the lymph moving freely and easily throughout your body.

Letting the lymphatic system become stagnant leads to impaired immunity and a degenerative process because the body is not able to properly cleanse and replenish.

Burning your rubbish

We accumulate waste in our body fat and the more fat we have, the more waste we collect.

What's more, once you have excess body fat, it becomes metabolically active itself, pumping out excess hormones that wreak as much internal havoc as many environmental toxins.

Exercise helps to reduce your risk by burning fat. When you burn fat, you not only release stored toxins into the bloodstream, where they can be filtered and excreted by your liver, kidneys and lungs, but you also eliminate the storage space where toxins hide.

Drink lots of water If you're exercising regularly, you're burning lots of fat and releasing stored toxins. So be sure to flush them from your system faster by also drinking plenty of fluids. Water helps to dilute and eliminate all those toxins; doctors suggest drinking 8 to 10 glasses of water per day, every day, but especially when you're exercising.

Sweating it out

You are wrapped in one of nature's finest waste-removal systems: your skin. The average adult has 1.6sq. m (18–20sq. ft) of skin. It weighs over 2.2kg (5lb), and though it doesn't look like a liver or a kidney, it is an excellent eliminative organ.

Like the liver and lungs, the skin excretes great amounts of metabolic waste and pollutants. Hence the phrase, 'sweat it out'.

Sweating is an excellent way of eliminating toxins. As you heat the body and perspire, you release heavy metals such as lead and mercury, organic toxins such as pesticides and insecticides, and various pollutants.

Though any heart-pumping aerobic exercise will work, there are special exercises designed to promote profuse sweating and detoxification.

Try hot yoga Bikram yoga, for example, is practiced in heated rooms with temperatures ranging from 29°C to 40°C (84°F to 104°F). This warm environment, combined with a vigorous routine that consists of 26 challenging poses, raises your heart rate and elicits sweat by the bucketful.

Bake a little Sitting in a sauna after exercise encourages even more elimination. (But you wouldn't want to do this right after Bikram yoga, however. That would be too much of a good thing. Never do more than you feel is right.)

Don't soak in your own toxins Wear workout clothes made from absorbent fabrics to pull the sweat away from your skin, and take a shower as soon as you can when you have finished exercising; you don't want those toxins sitting on your skin or being absorbed back in.

A clean sweep

Our bowel function has been described as 'Nature's broom'. Another big benefit of exercise is that it speeds metabolism and assists movement through the gut, keeping you regular, allowing for consistent waste removal.

Many people think you need enemas and colonics for detoxification, but in most cases, regular exercise is all the stimulation that your gastro-intestinal tract needs.

Physical activity also promotes increased circulation in general, which increases healthy bloodflow through important detoxifying organs like the kidneys and liver.

The key here is moderate exercise, which brings plenty of oxygen-rich blood to the organs and helps with the transfer of waste. Intense exercise won't have the same effect because blood tends to be shunted away from the abdominal area and into the working muscles during hard physical activity.

Both moderate and vigorous exercise help to blow out the cobwebs and clear your blood vessels and lungs, however. Sedentary people use only about one-third of their lung capacity. The other two-thirds contains stagnant air that is rich in toxins and metabolic waste. This not only prevents your lungs from doing their job properly, but it also limits the amount of oxygen-rich blood the rest of your body receives.

When you get your lungs huffing and puffing through physical activity, you blow the toxins from your lungs and allow more oxygen into your bloodstream. Many toxins can be broken into exhalable forms and expelled through increased respiration. So get moving!

Building your immunity team

One of the most important ways in which exercise helps to detoxify the body is by stimulating the immune system to build its arsenal of disease-fighting cells. These metabolic warriors (such as natural killer T cells and macrophages) patrol your body and neutralize harmful invaders before they can do their dirty work.

Exercise-immunology is an entire new field of medicine that focuses heavily on how exercise directly affects the immune system. We know regular, moderate exercise such as walking, jogging, cycling and swimming has a positive effect on many immune functions. Even short bursts of activity, throughout the day, will help.

A robust immune system is not only essential for keeping your system free from infection-causing viruses and bacteria, but it also plays a role in preventing cancer. Our immune system is always in surveillance mode, whether we exercise or not, but if you add exercise, it works even harder, and you're much less likely to get ill.

Curbing your stress

Lastly, but no less importantly, exercise helps with purification by purging toxic emotions. If it sounds 'New Agey' to talk about emotional pollution, consider this: stress – a runaway emotion in our society – causes a cascade of physical reactions including accelerated heartbeat, a rise in blood pressure, an increase in blood sugar and a boost in stomach acid.

Common symptoms of stress include muscle tension, upset stomach, headaches, fatigue, insomnia and compulsive eating, drinking or smoking – all of which not only hamper detoxification, but also pour more poison into your already-overworked system. Making matters worse, hormones like cortisol and adrenaline, which are associated with stress, promote fat (and thereby toxin) storage, particularly in the abdominal area.

Stress, hostility, and anger are well-established as serious risk factors for heart disease, and they are likely to contribute to other degenerative conditions as well.

Exercise provides stress-relief by burning off stress hormones and lowering blood pressure. Regular physical activity also makes you more stress-resilient.

Experts say the rigours of physical activity help the body to respond to all types of stress and ultimately protect the heart.

Exercise prescription

There are as many different types of exercise as there are ways you can imagine to move your body. Whether you run, dance, play sports, hop up and down on one foot, or even just lie on the floor and do roll-ups, it's all considered exercise. You might even dig out an old skipping rope.

Though all types of exercise will help you to detoxify, some are clearly more beneficial than others. Here are some for you to consider.

Walk this way

Generally speaking, aerobic exercises such as walking, jogging, cycling and swimming are the most detoxifying. You move the lymphatic system, you sweat, and you increase blood circulation and respiration.

Of the wide array of aerobic activities you can choose from, walking is the most popular. Almost everyone can do it, regardless of age or fitness levels, to get a daily dose of detoxification.

Walking energetically, planting on your heel and rocking up and pressing off of your toes with each step for about 20 minutes a day, is one of the easiest ways to stimulate your lymphatic system.

Jump for joy

Bouncing on a trampoline, such as a mini-trampoline or 'rebounder', is one of the least appreciated exercises for cleansing and strengthening every cell of your body. It's also one of the best workouts for activating the lymphatic system. Skipping is a great help, too.

Your lymphatic system is filled with millions of one-way valves that allow lymph to flow in one direction, usually upward. The change of speed and direction with each bounce opens every valve and gives your lymphatic system a super squeeze, so your cells are completely flushed of their metabolic waste and then saturated with incoming fresh oxygen and nutrients.

What's more, bouncing strengthens your muscles and bones, which respond to the increased force by getting stronger.

Many fitness centres have mini-trampolines available for general use. You can buy one at a sporting goods or department store or you can trawl the Internet for a supplier.

Let your body flow

Yoga is one of the few forms of exercise that can boast 5,000 years of faithful practice by millions of people across the globe. For centuries, it has been prescribed as moving medicine for the immune system. Yoga helps to lower stress hormones that compromise immunity while stimulating the lymphatic system to purge toxins and bringing fresh, nutrient-filled, oxygenated blood to each organ to ensure optimum function.

Yoga even includes specific poses that are believed to clear toxins from specific body regions and support specific body functions and organs. For instance, inverted poses like Downward Facing Dog (p. 95), which position your head and torso lower than other parts of your body, help to flush out your lungs and sinuses, so your body can oust bacteria and toxins caught in your mucus.

Whole-body stretching and strengthening exercises like yoga and tai chi are great detoxifiers because they stretch out the areas surrounding the lymph nodes through their full range of motion, and they encourage lymphatic drainage.

The gentle twisting, turning, bending, and reaching of mind-body exercises like yoga also put light pressure on your digestive system, which aids in the expulsion of toxins through your bowels.

Pick up the pace

There's a long-standing myth among exercisers that you need to exercise at a lower intensity for a longer duration to maximize fat burning and thereby release toxins. To really rev your metabolism, burn more calories, and keep your fat-burning switch turned on for a longer time after you have finished exercising, try picking up the pace a little.

Research shows that not only do you burn more calories when you exercise vigorously, but following the workout you get a robust hormonal charge that causes your body to burn more fat when you're at rest. What's more, your metabolism stays revved up five times longer after a spirited workout session than after an easy one. Over time, this can add up to burning an additional 100 to 200 calories a day, many of them from fat.

Slip in some fast time You don't have to imitate Olympic gold medallist Kelly Holmes, just sneak brief spurts of intensity into the aerobic workouts you already do. For instance, if you walk now, try picking up your pace and power walking or jogging just enough so that your breathing becomes heavy (but you're not gasping for breath) for 2 or 3 minutes. Then walk easy for 2 or 3 minutes. And so on. Before long, the higher-intensity segments will feel easier, and you'll be a speedier walker, too, so you'll be burning more calories each time you exercise.

Make some muscle

Sometime in our mid to late thirties, due to hormonal changes and generally decreasing activity levels, we start losing lean muscle tissue at the rate of about 0.25kg (8oz) a year – a loss that can accelerate to 0.5kg (1lb) a year in women once they hit menopause. That's important because muscle tissue burns about 15 times as many calories each day, even when you're just sleeping or reading, as fat tissue does.

When you lose muscle, your daily calorie burn drops. If you do nothing to stem the loss, by the time you're 65, you could have lost half of your lean body mass and doubled it with body fat. As you know, the more fat you have, the more room there is for toxins to hide out.

The best way to solve this problem is strength training, which boosts natural muscle-making chemicals such as human growth hormone and preserves the muscle we have, while also helping replace the muscle tissue we've lost.

Lifting weights also helps you to shed fat by burning calories. A 63.5kg (10 stone) woman can burn off almost 200 calories during a

WARNING Don't start a programme of strength training without first consulting your doctor.

challenging 30-minute strength-training routine. What's more, your calorie-burning metabolism can stay elevated for up to 48 hours after you've finished lifting.

Start lifting The key to maximizing your fat-burning metabolism is challenging as many muscle fibres as possible. That means starting a strength-training routine if you've never lifted weights before, or changing your routine to a new, more challenging one if you have.

Target as many muscles as you can The more muscles you recruit in your lifting routine, the more lean tissue and the less toxin-trapping fat you'll have. A woman who targets all her major muscle groups twice a week can expect to replace 2.25kg (5lb) of muscle – five to ten years' worth – in just a few months of strength training.

Take it outside

Whenever possible, infuse your exercise routine with some fresh air by exercising outdoors, ideally going somewhere beautiful like a park, along a river, by the ocean or into the mountains.

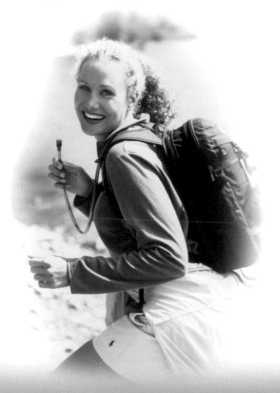

Even if you just walk down a tree-lined street, however, you're still helping your body to detoxify and heal. Human beings have a natural affinity with the outdoors. One much-cited study from the mid-1980s demonstrated that people recovering from abdominal surgery with a view of nature from their windows had significantly shorter hospital stays, required less pain medication and made fewer complaints than those whose rooms faced a brick wall. And, of course, plants and trees help to detoxify us by filtering our air and cleansing our environment of carbon dioxide and other environmental pollutants.

When exercising outside, however, it's important that you do not add to your toxic burden by walking or jogging along crowded roads where you're breathing exhaust. This is particularly important in warm-weather months, when the pollution tends to get trapped in the atmosphere, clogging the air we breathe with heavy metals and other dangerous elements. It's even more important if you're doing a spirited exercise like jogging or cycling that increases your breathing rate. When exercising vigorously, your air intake increases tenfold. And most of the air is getting pulled right through your mouth, which, unlike your nose, isn't lined with fine hairs that filter the air before it reaches your lungs.

To avoid nullifying your detoxifying exercise with environmental pollutants, exercise at the right time and place. Some simple tips:

Avoid the rush Avoid exercising during morning and evening rush hours. If you must exercise at that time of day, get as far away from the roads as you can to avoid direct exposure.

Shed and scrub Pollutants collect on your clothes and skin when you exercise. Change clothes and hop in the shower (or at least towel off) as soon as possible when you've finished.

Check the index Most TV, newspaper and online weather reports give an air pollution level forecast, especially when highs are expected.

Chapter 6
Fasting and cleansing
Lightening your body's toxic burden

No matter how well you eat, you are exposed to – and take into your body – a variety of chemical toxins that humans have never before had to deal with during our millennia-long evolutionary journey.

It's no surprise that our bodies get gummed up. Toxins build up in the liver, kidneys and blood; they get stored away in the fat and they may end up contributing to awful degenerative diseases like cancer and heart disease. They also contribute to the ageing process. All good reasons to get rid of as much of your toxic overload as possible.

That leads to one of the main concerns that needs to be addressed up front, before we look at the benefits of fasting and cleansing and how to go about it. Practitioners of alternative medicine have prescribed fasting and cleansing therapies for decades – actually for centuries, if you consider the traditional practices of India and the Orient. As alternative medicine becomes more widespread and people learn about the outstanding benefits that fasting and cleansing can provide, they've responded with enthusiasm – sometimes with a little too much enthusiasm.

They reason that if a little fasting is good, a lot must be better. If a little cleansing is good, why not really push the boat out and then go for a good, long fast? For a lot of reasons, that's not a good idea – at least not if you're contemplating doing this on your own, without medical supervision.

Health practitioners use fasting as one of many healing modalities that also include nutrition, meditation, massage and exercise.

Most people are nutritionally deficient and when they fast, they disturb their body. If your regular daily eating habits are not already healthy, you'd be better off concentrating your efforts on improving your daily diet, and putting off any thoughts of fasting until you've succeeded.

If you're not properly prepared before you fast, your body will not only not detoxify, it will think it's starving and respond by holding onto everything it has – including the toxins. You'll feel irritated, headachy and exhausted. And your metabolism will slow down. Then, once you start

WARNING

Some people should not fast at all. These include:

• Women who are pregnant or nursing.

• Young children.

• People who are extremely thin or who have eating disorders.

• People who have diabetes, cancer, heart disease or any other serious illness. These people should not do even short fasts on their own. While they may benefit from fasting, they should do so only under the close supervision of a health care professional experienced in supervising therapeutic fasts.

to eat again, you'll feel compelled to gorge and will likely gain weight. And, after all that work you've done, you'll still be carrying the toxic load that is stressing your body and threatening your health.

Learn how to live well all the time: don't just pollute yourself, then do a cleansing a couple of times a year. Support your cleansing organs every day. Breathe deeply, eat correctly, sweat, take liver-cleansing herbs.

If you do all of these things your body will be ready to benefit from its first fast. If you don't do these things on a regular basis, there's a good chance that fasting will be not only unpleasant, but also not particularly helpful.

Preparing to fast

You can get your body used to the idea of fasting by doing a small fast every single day. Every evening at 7pm, stop eating and fast until breakfast. Let your body do its cleanse and repair.

Your body uses an incredible amount of energy (and nutrients) digesting its food. If you spend the evening snacking without ever giving your body a chance to empty your stomach and move things along, you're adding to your toxic load.

It's fine to have a cup of herbal tea while you're watching TV or reading in the evening, but you really should train yourself to stop eating after dinner. That will accomplish more detoxification on an ongoing basis than fasting a couple of times a year.

Fasting basics

If you want to further enhance your body's cleanup efforts, a certain amount of fasting is helpful, provided the fasts are short, supported by adequate nutrition and conducted safely. Here's an overview of the basic procedure for conducting a fast, no matter what its length:
- Prepare your body to fast.
- Leave stress behind.
- Start slowly. Don't try a longer fast until your body has learned how to benefit from shorter fasts.
- Unless you're conducting a longer therapeutic fast under medical supervision, give your body enough nutrition to support the fasting process.
- At all times, put safety first.
- Come out of your fast carefully and with the right kind of nutritional support.

Getting started

To begin, be very clear about the benefits that you hope to gain from fasting. If you're not clear on what you hope to gain, you'll find that your resolve will disappear at the first hunger pang. Here are ways to prepare for a fast:

Adjust your diet Before you fast, set a date a week or so away, and begin to lighten up your diet.

Focus on fibre Make sure you eat plenty of high-fibre foods, fruits and vegetables in the days leading up to your fast. Enjoy plenty of fresh juices every day for several days before you fast.

Get hydrated Drink plenty of water. Aim for at least eight glasses a day.

Be a little stricter with yourself If you haven't already done so as part of your regular diet, now is the time to cut right back on meats, sugar and fatty foods.

Keep moving Get plenty of exercise. At the very least, go for a walk every day.

Ease in slowly

Don't just jump right into a three-day fast. If you've never fasted before, try skipping the occasional meal, replacing what you'd normally eat with a glass of freshly prepared (not canned or bottled) fruit or vegetable juice.

Do a couple of practice fasts After you've tried skipping a meal a few times, try fasting for just a single day, a few times.

Give your body time to adjust As your body learns to benefit from a short fast, it will co-operate by starting to release its toxic overload as soon as it feels the fasting routine that you've established get underway.

Pick up the pace After you've done a couple of one-day fasts, you can try a longer fast, anywhere from two to three days, on your own. Fasts that are any longer than that really fall under the category of medical therapy and should be undertaken only under the supervision of a trained health care professional. Your health could be compromised, as could your ability to think clearly. Have someone at least monitor what you're doing. Don't self-treat.

Pamper yourself If you've never fasted before, you probably don't want your first time to be during your working week. Pick a weekend or, better yet, a three-day weekend, when you can pamper yourself. Spend some time going for walks in beautiful surroundings, writing a diary or listening to music.

Take advantage of this special time Many traditions use fasting as part of spiritual discipline, and some people find that even a fast of a few days proves to be a time of unusual mental clarity and alertness. If you're not ready to fast or you're overdoing it, fasting can have an unpleasant side effect – mental fog.

Even if your fast is entirely for physical, detoxification reasons, this can be a special time to relax and turn your thoughts inward.

Nutrition while fasting

By strict definition, a fast means doing without food entirely and subsisting on just water. But the word 'fasting' has come to be used to cover a whole range of dietary regimes that eliminate regular meals. This can mean 'fasting' on just one food, or fasting by skipping a couple of meals and replacing them with a simple food like dry toast or juice.

Many health fasting experts now recommend doing exactly that – taking in a modest number of nutrients while otherwise fasting.

Here's how to give your body a reasonable amount of nutritional support while fasting:

Limit yourself to a simple dish Try fasting either on fresh juices or, if you find that too rigorous, try limiting your meals to one simple, nutritious dish. A favourite is a simple Indian dish of beans and rice known as kichari. (See the recipe for Fenugreek kichari on page 107). For most people, freshly made fruit or vegetable juice is the alternative that's best for the body.

One technique that works nicely for many people is to have fresh juices for breakfast and dinner and have kichari for lunch. If you give your body simple nutrition, it's easier to release toxins. The purpose of a fast is to help your body to unburden itself without strain.

Get juiced For people who are accustomed to fasting, try drinking freshly made fruit and vegetable juices every couple of hours during the day – or days – of fasting. Have orange juice in the morning, then later in the day switch to other kinds of juice – such as carrot, celery, parsley, tomato or cucumber.

Enjoy taste and variety There are a number of juicing recipes beginning on page 128, and there are also great recipes for fresh juices both online and in recipe books devoted solely to juicing. And if you're fasting during the winter, you can make hot vegetable broths. Simply use your favourite vegetables to make soup, then strain.

Carrots, cabbage, parsley and onions are all good choices. Juices are absorbed readily and are an easy source of nutrition. They're low in calories, but they provide enough nutrition to both support the detoxification process and to help your body to understand that it's not starving, so it can begin to release its toxic load.

Have an exit strategy

When you fast, your body closes down its production of the enzymes and other biochemicals that you need to digest your food. And unless you return to eating in a slow and methodical manner, you could end up with a mass of undigested food blocking your digestive system and releasing toxins back into your cleaned-up body.

You need to back out of a juice-only fast as carefully as you eased into it. On the day you choose to end your fast, have a little fresh fruit for breakfast and lunch and dinner. The next day, have some steamed vegetables or a salad for lunch and dinner. The day after, you can add a cereal or a meal made with whole grains. The idea is to let your body get 'warmed up' again before it has to deal with solid meals.

Ending a fast quickly

If you're in the middle of what you thought was going to be a three-day fast and you find that you can't go on, just have a piece of fruit. Or, if you're really uncomfortable, make yourself a bowl of oatmeal or a baked potato. Your unpleasant symptoms should disappear almost immediately. One thing you should not do at this point is either overeat or reach for an unhealthy food.

Fasting and cleansing have become so trendy that many well-meaning but inadequately trained people are happy to supervise your fast for a fee. If you're going to try a longer fast under supervision, talk to your doctor first.

And if someone tells you to go on because your unpleasant fasting symptoms are only a 'healing crisis' (see pages 17 and 58), use your own judgement. It is possible to have a healing crisis while you're detoxifying your body, but there are ways to detoxify that do not involve nausea or delirium. It's alright to end a fast any time your body tells you that you've had enough.

Longer fasts: serious therapy

Fasting over an extended period of time can be an effective healing therapy – both extended modified fasts and fasting on just water have been used for centuries, and people keep on using them for healing purposes because they work.

It is important to provide nutritional support both for the liver and for the other detoxifying systems of the body. If all these systems need nutrients in order to do their jobs, then how can extended fasting or fasting on just water for any length of time be effective? How can detoxification, not to mention alleviation of disease symptoms, even take place?

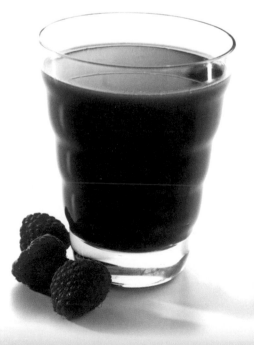

LISTEN TO YOUR BODY

When your body begins throwing off its excess toxins, they have to come out somewhere. They leave their places of storage via your bloodsteam, your liver, your kidneys, your lungs and the very pores of your skin. And depending upon how much comes out and how fast, they can create unpleasant symptoms. These include:

- Abdominal discomfort
- Anxiousness
- Assorted body aches
- Bad breath
- Body odour
- Dizziness

- Headaches
- Insomnia
- Irritability
- Mental fogginess
- Nausea

You can safely put up with a mild level of discomfort and be the judge of how much discomfort you're willing to experience in order to give your body a chance to detoxify. But there are a couple of symptoms that should automatically signal the end of a fast:

- Abdominal pain
- Delirium
- Emotional or psychological distress
- Fever

- Heart palpitations or irregularities
- Vomiting
- Watery diarrhoea

Watery diarrhoea can cause the body to lose electrolytes, important minerals that the body needs in order to perform certain functions, such as keeping the heart beating. In general, pay attention to how you feel and respect what your body is trying to tell you. If you're feeling so uncomfortable that you're questioning the wisdom of fasting in the first place, just end the fast.

Fasting is not an endurance test or a test of willpower, and should not be a cause for suffering. The kind of gentle fasts we're discussing here are for the purpose of detoxifying and cleansing your body. If you're carrying a heavy toxic load and you're cleaning out the toxins a little too swiftly, you're going to feel awful. The answer is to slow down. Go ahead and end the fast but continue eating a healthy diet for a time. And, if you're so inclined, try a shorter fast at some point in the future. Don't feel that you've failed. Simply acknowledge that you've listened to your body and move on.

HERBAL CLEANSING KITS

No matter what kind of fast you're on – short, long, mono-diet, juice, water only – there are herbs that can help to support and expedite your cleanse. Many of these herbs were described in Chapter 4.

There are also numerous kits that you can buy, either in health food stores or online, that can prove helpful. These typically consist of a bulking agent, usually psyllium, plus herbs that encourage bowel movements and support your liver and other cleansing systems of your body. You may even choose probiotics, strains of friendly bacteria intended to prevent the toxic kind from taking up residence in your cleaned-out gut. While these kits are fairly expensive it's convenient to have all cleansing supplies packaged together along with a schedule and dietary recommendations.

If you opt for a kit and experience watery diarrhoea, muscle spasms or both, use less of the product. Discontinue its use altogether if the unpleasant side-effects don't disappear.

There's no disputing the fact that people with chronic illnesses who have not been helped by anything else may experience dramatic improvements when they fast for extended periods of time. To be effective, these fasts can be on just water and they can last for many days. But they absolutely must be under medical supervision. Research suggests impressive results with a wide variety of conditions such as:

- Arthritis
- Asthma
- Depression
- Diabetes
- Fibroids
- Heart disease
- High blood pressure
- Irritable bowel syndrome
- Lupus, as well as many other autoimmune diseases
- Mental illness, including schizophrenia
- Obesity
- Skin conditions, including acne, eczema and psoriasis
- Ulcers

Most specialists say the best results have come from fasts of approximately one week.

Following a fast, some people with suspected food allergies do a 'food challenge'; that is, they reintroduce suspect foods one at a time in order to determine which foods are problematic. Foods you are allergic or sensitive to are the potential culprits in a whole host of chronic and painful conditions.

People who are planning to detoxify as a means of dealing with chronic diseases should not try fasting on their own. This is really important. Only undertake fasting under medical supervision.

If you have a chronic condition that might respond to fasting and you'd like to try it, you need to find a health care professional who is experienced in conducting therapeutic fasts.

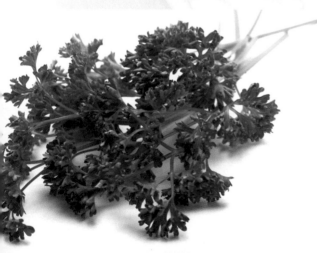

Flushing the toxic colon

We can't leave the subject of fasting and cleansing without taking a look at the whole area of enemas and colonics. Both techniques involve physically flushing the colon with warm water.

Enemas are self-administered, using an inexpensive piece of equipment – a bag that looks like a hot water bottle, with a tube and nozzle.

Colonics are administered in a clinical setting by a professional. The difference is that the apparatus that delivers the colonic makes it possible to refill and flush several times for a more thorough cleansing, and it goes much further up into the body.

The jury is still out on whether colonic washing during and following a fast is necessary or even useful. Enemas and colonics do have enthusiastic proponents who feel that these techniques are an important part of fasting.

Most of us could use some help with colon cleansing, especially if bowel movements are sluggish. But during a fast, the body is throwing off lots of toxic material. This comes out through the lungs, through sweat, through urine, and through stools.

A daily self-administered enema during a fast. and a couple of colonics toward the end of a fast are recommended by some practioners.

If you choose to do this, keep a few things in mind for your safety:

Don't overdo it No more than one enema a day. If you do, you could absorb too much water and throw your electrolyte balance off.

Use standard equipment It is possible to do damage with too much water pressure. And follow to the letter the directions on the package that the enema equipment comes in.

Keep it to yourself Don't share equipment with other family members. Make sure you clean the nozzle thoroughly after each use. Soak it in bleach and water to properly clean it.

Don't use tap water You don't want to absorb things like chlorine and other toxic substances found in water direct from the tap. Use bottled, filtered or distilled water, instead.

Put safety first Enemas can make you feel depleted. If you are elderly or have certain chronic diseases, such as diabetes, uncontrolled high blood pressure or congestive heart failure, never self-administer an enema. In these cases, enemas can be safely used only under the advice and supervision of a professional.

And here's what to look for if you're opting for a series of colonics:

Find the right professional Your best bet is to get a referral from a doctor, naturopath or other health care professional whom you know and trust. Alternatively, inquire about the training and experience of the person who will be administering the colonics. Do be aware that inadequately trained people can do serious damage to the bowel.

Insist on cleanliness Make sure that the clinic uses disposable specula and tubing.

Ask about the water. If the clinic uses tap water rather than filtered water in their machines, simply go elsewhere.

Don't get taken for a ride It's fine to have a series of colonics over several weeks, but don't let someone talk you into coming back week after week on into the future.

Finally, we should take a look at a couple of cleansing techniques that are a lot easier to use and are quite effective. You'll benefit greatly by adding these into your daily routine for the rest of your life.

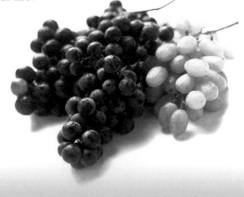

Floss & scrape

You may not think brushing and flossing your teeth are an important way to detoxify your body, but they are.

Your mouth as a haven for bacteria – a nice, warm, moist environment with plenty of food, where they can, and do, multiply. You brush your teeth in the morning and just a few hours later, when you run your tongue over your teeth, you feel a film. That's not saliva; that's the toxic outer coating (glycocalyx) of bacteria that multiply in your mouth.

Bacteria that grow in your mouth don't just cause bad breath. The type responsible for gum disease has been implicated as one possible cause of heart disease, as well. So you really do want to brush and floss them out daily.

In addition, consider a tongue scraper. These come in all kinds of shapes and are readily available in chemists and health food stores. (You don't have to get a fancy one – a clean teaspoon will do just as well.) Some toothbrushes have a scraper built in to the back of the head. Once you've finished brushing and flossing, swipe the scraper over your tongue a couple of times and you'll dislodge a few million more toxic bacteria.

Say 'Hello' to neti

If you grew up in a different culture – India's, to be exact – there's a good chance you'd clean the inside of your nose too. And if you regularly have problems with sinusitis or allergies to pollens, dust, mould, pet dander and so on, or if you're the first in your office to catch a cold, you might want to consider a daily nasal wash with a neti pot.

Every day we breathe in particles, dirt, germs, and pollution. They stick to the mucous membrane in the back of the throat. If you wash the particles away, you have less of a chance of getting sick or reacting to them.

Your nose is lined with tiny hairs that serve to block particles. And the mucous membrane at the back of your throat are made of cells covered with tiny hairlike structures. These living hairs (cilia) work in unison to push any pollutants back out through the nose or down your throat to your stomach, where the dirt is eliminated.

In a dry climate (including everyone's heated house in winter) or in a dusty or polluted environment, the mucous membrane gets dried out, or the mucus thickens and builds up. Then these tiny cilia are easily overpowered and can't do their job of protecting you. Hence plugged-up sinuses, often followed by sinus headaches.

You can clear up sinus problems by using a neti pot (which resembles a small teapot) to pour warm, salty water through your nose. It takes only a minute or two each day for the neti pot to draw excess mucus out of your nasal passages and cleanse them thoroughly of accumulated dust and pollutants.

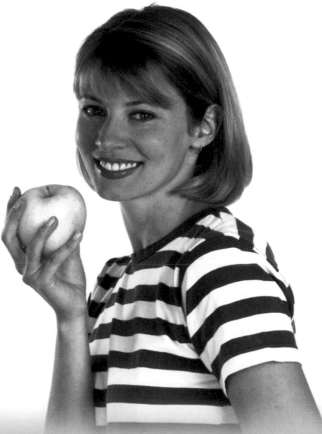

HOW TO USE A NETI POT

1 **Get inspired** The first time you see someone use a neti pot, you'll be amazed that it's possible to pour water into one nostril and have it come out the other. The key is to position your head correctly. You'll need to read through the directions and get a sense of how it works. The water simply pours right through without causing any discomfort. It won't go down your throat unless you raise your head and let it go down. Once you get over feeling that it's a weird thing to do, it becomes so routine it's like brushing your teeth.

2 **Prepare the pot** Dissolve ½ to ⅔ of a teaspoon of sea salt in 1½ cups of warm water. This is enough water to fill the pot twice and do both nostrils. You use sea salt because it's pure. You don't want to stick the typical additives in table salt – iodine or anti-caking agents such as sodium silico-aluminate – up your nose. And the water should be about as comfortably warm as bath water. Now fill the neti pot.

3 **Position your head** Stand over your bathroom basin with your face looking directly down into the basin. Then tilt your head so that your right nostril is higher than your left. Now insert the spout of the pot into your right nostril and pour. The water will pour directly through and come out of your left nostril, bringing with it excess mucus along with any dust and pollutants that have lodged inside your nose.

4 **Expel excess water** Blow your nose gently. There's a lot of liquid to get rid of and if you use excessive pressure, you could end up with liquid in your eustachian tubes – the little internal tubes that connect your throat to your ears. If you do this, you'll have a clogged sensation in your ears. The water will drain out of its own accord after a while, but you can avoid this unpleasantness by blowing gently.

5 **Repeat on the other side** Tip your head so your left nostril is higher than your right, and pour a second pot of salted water through in the other direction.

6 **Adjust your recipe for comfort** The water pouring through your nostrils should create a pleasant sensation. If you feel any discomfort, it's for one of two reasons:

• The water temperature isn't right. The water really needs to be pleasantly warm. If you pour cold water or water that's too hot into your nose, it hurts. The idea is to use body-temperature water. Your nasal passages deal with warm liquids all the time.

• The salt content isn't right. Adjust the salt content slightly the next time you mix the solution.

After a while, you'll get a sense of the right temperature and the salt concentration that's best for you. For a short video that demonstrates the technique, you can visit the Neti Pot Company web site at *www.bytheplanet.com/Products/ Yoga/neti/Netipot.htm.*

Chapter 7
Pure mind, pure heart
Detoxing your emotions and moods

We all have our superstitions — certain habits, ways of thinking, moods, dilemmas and negative emotional moments that seem to bring us bad luck. Overcoming or controlling them is an important part of your detox.

Our negative emotions can become pervasive, affecting not only how we feel but also our physical health, mental outlook, relationships with others, families, careers, even digestion and sleep patterns. That's why it's so important to identify and get rid of them.

The techniques of emotional detoxification described briefly here come from many different religious, cultural and scientific traditions.

Take stress, as an example — even brief psychological stress can produce changes in your heartbeat and adrenaline levels while reducing your immune response. There's also a link between stress, depression and common illnesses like colds and flu.

Prayer for health & healing

Many researchers have been studying the power of a variety of spiritual, religious, psychological and mental experiences to improve our outlook and our health. It appears that people who pray can help to alleviate conditions such as high blood pressure, headaches and anxiety. What's more, prayer has been shown to speed the healing of wounds and even recovery from heart attacks. Even the level of red blood cells in your body can be affected by prayer.

Relax to detox

Many of us have a fight-or-flight response to numerous experiences in everyday life — with pumping adrenaline, soaring blood pressure and accelerated breathing. To counterbalance these moments, there is the relaxation response. There are many ways to induce this response but whatever you choose to do, you will become less frenetic, so your metabolism (the rate at which you burn energy) decreases. So does muscle tension. Your blood pressure, heart rate and breathing rate all become modulated.

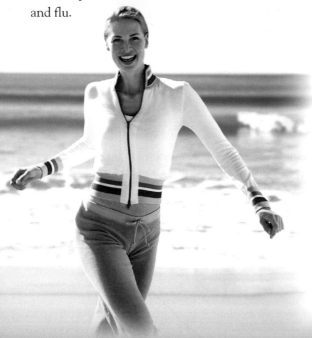

Cleansing breaths

Many spiritual traditions make use of a variety of breathing techniques. These can help you to focus, reduce stress and cleanse yourself of unnecessary fear and agitation.

Observe your breath cycle Sitting in a comfortable position with your eyes closed and clothing loosened, breathe normally as you pay close attention to your breathing. Do this for about 3 minutes.

Focus on exhalation Every time you exhale, try to squeeze more and more air out of your lungs. Your inhalations will also deepen, but that happens automatically, because the more air you force out, the more you have to take in.

Let yourself be 'breathed' Lie on your back and imagine that you are passively receiving the breath that passes through you. With each exhalation, air is being sucked out of you, and with each inhalation, the breath is being blown into you. Try to hold on to this perception for ten breaths. It's an exercise you can do nightly before you fall asleep.

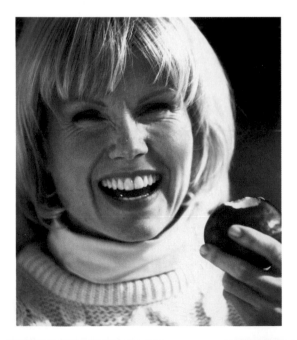

The purifying power of laughter

It has been proved, scientifically, that laughter is good for you. Researchers have found that stress decreases and immunity increases among those who have the strongest humour response. So try to laugh more, tell jokes and see the funny side of life.

Manage your time and territory

If you feel as if you are in a state of constant disorganization and confusion, stress can take a heavy toll. Here are two ways that experts recommend to help you to get your family organized, your activities on schedule and your papers in order.

Create a family calendar Once a week, get together with everyone in your household and go over the weekly calendar so you don't have any surprises during the week. Get everyone to check it every morning.

Assign a purpose to every piece of paper Paper tends to pile up, often because we can't figure out whether to keep it, throw it away or file it somewhere. You can simplify the process if you put every piece of paper (or the information it contains) into one of several places.

- A 'to sort' tray
- The waste paper basket
- Into your calendar
- On your 'to do' list
- Into an action file
- Into a personal phone book or file of telephone numbers
- Into a reference file

DEFUSING ROAD RAGE

In moments of anger, blood pressure rises, metabolism increases and we're at increased risk of heart attack and stroke. But apart from the physical cost, anger can lead to life-threatening behaviour, particularly if you happen to be driving a car.

The most effective way to deal with anger involves two basic approaches: relaxation exercises and what's called cognitive relaxation therapy. Both approaches are effective, especially when used in combination. Here's how you can deal with road rage before it happens.

Extend your breathing Suppose someone just swerved in front of you, nearly causing an accident. Internally, you experience this incident as a life-threatening situation, and your body reacts as if you have to fight for your life. Immediately you start to breathe faster. But stop right there! Concentrate on expelling all the air from your lungs, then take a deep breath. No matter what you're thinking or how angry you're feeling, just concentrate on your slow, deep breaths.

Tense and relax your body If you're driving, you can't jump up and down to help dispel anger. But you'll get a similar effect if you consciously tense and release the muscles in different parts of your body, particularly the areas that tense up when you're angry. This can be done without moving very much at all. Tighten the muscles around your neck and shoulders, hold for a moment, then relax. Then tighten and relax your arm muscles. Then do your stomach muscles. As you move through your body, progressively tensing and relaxing, you can still concentrate on driving. But you'll find that when you have finished, the nervous energy generated by your anger has been dispersed.

Have a chat with yourself If you want to, you can consciously change your thinking. For instance, if a car is on your tail, you might have an angry impulse to speed up ('Okay, mate, let's see how fast you want to go!') or slow down ('If you insist on tailgating, I'll just stay in your way.'). You can actually replace these thoughts if you talk to yourself and say, 'I'm going at the right speed, and I'll continue at this speed. I hope you don't take the risk of passing me, but if you decide to do that, there's nothing I can do to prevent you.'

If you can change your thought pattern, you can prevent a bad situation from becoming worse.

Office tactics for stress relief

Here are some simple progressive relaxation techniques that you can do at work without stirring from your seat. Try to remain focused during the brief periods when you're doing these exercises. If you make a habit of doing these exercises every hour or so, after two weeks they will become habitual. Then you can actually prevent stress, rather than react to it.

Trigger some relaxation Sitting relaxed in an upright position, take three deep, slow breaths while you relax the muscles of your head and face. Let your shoulders drop and release the tension from your neck muscles. (After the initial three deep breaths, resume breathing normally.)

Give tension an outlet Ball up your fists and tense the muscles all the way from your wrists up your arms to your biceps and shoulders. Hold the tension for a count of five, then release. As you release, visualize the blood smoothly flowing down into your arms, into your wrists, and all the way to your fingertips.

Pay attention to your legs and feet If you can, slip off your shoes and curl your toes. If that's not possible, just press down firmly on the balls of your feet. Tighten all the muscles of your lower legs, flexing your calves. Again, hold this pose for a count of five, then release and visualize the blood flowing all the way down to the tips of your toes, reviving your feet.

Hunch your shoulders high Hold for a count of five, then release and relax.

Make faces Finally, tighten and release the muscles of your face and forehead to ease the tension all around the facial area.

Getting through life's changes

In studies of stress, researchers have learned that any kind of significant change in life, positive as well as negative, can raise stress levels. To face such events, it helps to be prepared with some strategies to release the stress you feel. Here are some methods.

Count your blessings Whether you're going through times of great hardship or on the brink of something new and different, you can help your physical and emotional well-being if you realistically 'count your blessings'.

Smooth your move to a new home As soon as you are in, set up your bedroom before anything else. You'll feel far more relaxed, if you know you can retreat to that familiar area at day's end.

Use your answering machine Instead of jumping up immediately to answer the phone every time it rings, let your machine take the calls and answer them when it suits you.

Removing fears & phobias

Studies of disaster situations point to the conclusion that fear has a physical effect. To protect our bodies as well as our minds from the stress of fear, we need coping mechanisms. Here are some of the best.

Tap for relief Using a technique that combines physical distraction with mental prompting, you can help yourself to dispel fear and restore calm almost immediately. First think about the fear

MEDITATION TO RENEW YOUR MIND

Stop worrying . . . buoy your spirits . . . boost your pleasure! While these may sound like promises of a magic elixir or an illegal drug, they are actually the benefits of something we can all learn – meditation.

The purpose of meditation is simply to train your awareness to be in the moment. When you're lost in thoughts and emotions, you're dealing with the past and the future. By meditating, you can observe those thoughts and emotions instead of experiencing them.

Meditation teachers recommend that you focus on something very arbitrary and specific – your breathing, a phrase or a single word. For instance, you might try to focus on the single area of your nostrils where you feel the intake of breath. While maintaining that focus, your mind will naturally wander, but that doesn't matter. Gently bring your mind and your attention back to your breath. Do that without judging or blaming yourself.

that you have to deal with, while you try to evaluate (on a scale of 1 to 10) how fearful you're feeling. Then, using two fingers, tap firmly five times on the following points:

- About 2.5cm (1in) under the eye, high on the cheek
- About 10cm (4in) directly below the armpit
- About 2.5cm (1in) down and 2.5cm (1in) to the left or right of the centre collarbone notch
- The crown of the head
- The chin
- Both wrists

Each of these points corresponds to an acupuncture or acupressure point in Chinese medicine, where the *chi* (positive energy) is particularly concentrated. By tapping repeatedly at these points, you help to release the energy and distract yourself from fear.

Hum When you feel fearful, just hum or sing to yourself. This quick therapy works because the left side of your brain is the centre of emotions that create worry and fear. When you hum or sing, you activate the right side of your brain, which helps to overwhelm some of the nerve-jangling alarms that come from the left.

Have faith Associated with fear and anxiety is the dread that you might not survive what you're feeling. It can be reassuring to dwell on the fact that you've survived the fear before and you can do it again.

Whatever you do, keep breathing Part of the fight-or-flight reaction is hyperventilation. Without even knowing that it's happening, you tense up and take fast, shallow breaths when you feel fear. As your body becomes oxygen-deprived, it sends more panic signals, so the original fear is compounded by a primal fear of suffocation. It's important to break this cycle and avoid hyperventilation. You can learn to prevent it yourself, just by being aware of when fear is making you breathe more rapidly. Then slow down your breathing and try to pace yourself.

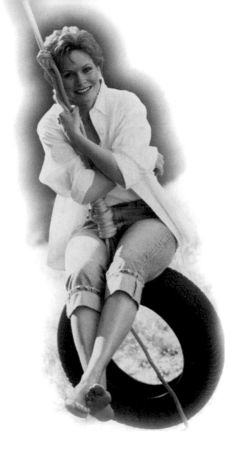

Detox your relationships

Disagreements and disputes can cast a long shadow. It's hard to feel good about a discussion that turns into an argument or a dispute that reaches boiling point. You can avoid the dynamics that lead to this kind of escalation with some rules that will help to prevent anger and defensiveness from poisoning a relationship.

Say how you feel It is far more effective and less likely to cause conflict if you use 'I' statements to get your point of view across. Sentences that start 'You always...' or 'You never...' are bound to make the situation worse.

Attack the problem, not the person To resolve conflicts amicably, focus on the issues and work together toward a solution. In the initial stage, you need to identify both what you and the other person want. Working together, generate a number of possible solutions, evaluate them and then decide on the best one.

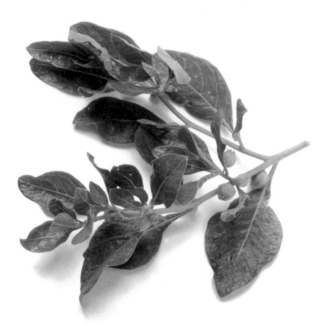

Mirror the other person's point of view Misunderstandings happen all too easily, especially when we feel as if we are being attacked or defied. One way to avoid mistaking a message is with a process called mirroring. That is, make sure you understand what the other person is trying to say, and let that person know you are listening before you try to respond.

Detox your new home

Your emotions are definitely affected by your home environment. If you move into a new house, office or flat, or even if you've lived in the same place for a long time, the atmosphere can feel wrong if something unpleasant has occurred there. You need to get rid of the 'bad vibes'.

Traditional practices of feng shui can be extremely helpful when it comes to detoxifying a space and replacing bad feelings with positive energy. The objective is to create an environment that allows the maximum flow of *chi* (positive energy) around the home. Many factors are involved, from the positioning of doors, windows and furniture to the arrangement of plants, pictures, lights, crystals and wind chimes. Because emotional energy is considered such a critical component of health and lifestyle, practitioners of feng shui pay special attention to areas of the home that can contribute to negative emotions such as betrayal, anger and despair.

Buy a book on feng shui cures and use them around your home or office.

Rituals for purifying moods & emotions

In your own detox programme, you may have discovered that your daily activities can be enhanced by introducing ritualistic or ceremonial qualities to everyday actions.

Washing your hands is a very ordinary activity, but it takes on a different quality if you are mindful of the warm water, use a soap with a pleasant fragrance, and gently massage the tension out of your hands while you're washing.

The following are three traditional ceremonies with special meaning within the culture they come from. Though they aren't from our culture, it is still possible to learn from them and adapt them to your own daily life.

A Mayan purifying bath

In Mayan tradition, ritual baths helped to rid the soul of the diseases associated with human suffering. Spiritual bathing practices were used to deal with fright, trauma, sadness, envy, grief and many other emotions. Certain herbs were associated with spiritual illnesses.

Many of the fresh herbs used by the Mayans are not readily available today. But there is a winter bath using dried herbs that can have the purifying effect of the ritual Mayan bath. You can use either a single dried herb or a combination of different

YOGA ROUTINE FOR DETOXING YOUR EMOTIONS

According to yoga tradition, many of your emotional responses are centred or focused in one particular area of your body – what's called the anahata chakra. Symbolized in drawings by a six-pointed star, this is the area that needs to be treated if you become excessively insecure, nervous, anxious or angry. The following is a simple yoga exercise that helps to bring awareness to the anahata chakra, producing a greater sense of well-being.

Assume the position Kneel on a rug or mat with your knees together, your shins flat on the floor, and your feet under your buttocks. Bend forward as far as you can. If possible, try to rest your stomach and chest on your thighs and your forehead on the floor, with your hands placed palms-down on either side of your head. If you are overweight, it's okay to let your knees come apart to allow space for your abdomen.

Move with your breath Inhale deeply and rise up, spreading your arms. At the height of the inhalation, your upper body should be straight and your gaze toward the ceiling. As you look up, raise your arms with your palms open.

Lower your arms Do this on the exhalation, bringing your palms down to cover your heart while you chant 'Yam'. This is a traditional chant word that allows for varied expression and intonation. When chanting, repeat the sound as often as you like, drawing out the 'a' sound in 'Yam', then closing your lips to produce a long, humming 'm' sound.

Co-ordinate your movements As you inhale again, raise your arms again to the open position. Exhale and return to the crouched, kneeling starting position.

Repeat one to eight times Chant 'Yam' every time you change from the upraised-arms position to the hands-on-heart position.

herbs, including basil, rosemary, sage, thyme, oregano and dried roses. The scent of rosemary is traditionally used to improve memory and relieve sorrow; the scent of sage helps to reduce fatigue; and the ever-popular rose is commonly used to treat stress and insomnia.

Conducting spiritual bathing at home is rewarding and easy. Here's how.

1 **Prepare ahead of time** Add 1 cup of dried herbs (use any of the above) to 4.5 litres (8 pints) of water, bring it all to the boil for 5 minutes, then turn off the heat and let the herbs steep for 1 hour.

2 **Strain out the herbs** When the herbal mixture has steeped and cooled, pour it through a strainer into a second 4.5 litre (8 pint) container, filtering out the loose herbs.

3 Prepare the bath Fill your bathtub with warm tap water and pour the herbal 'tea' into the tub.

4 Luxuriate in your bath. Soak, meditate and pray for at least half an hour, staying as relaxed as possible.

A Native American parting ritual

To begin the ritual, relatives and members of the tribe gather in a circle. Herbs are placed in a smudge pot or woven into braids tied with cotton string. Someone lights the herb, then blows out the flame. As it continues to smoke, the smoke is not inhaled, but with cupped hands, each person draws in some of the smoke toward his head, face or torso. As the smoke drifts away, it carries the prayers that mourners send to their ancestors.

According to tradition, as the smoke passes over different parts of the body, it has a variety of effects. Drawn toward the heart, it increases love. As it weaves around the face and head, it brings clearer vision. Swept over the limbs and torso, it has a relaxing effect, stripping away anger and stress. A feeling of peace descends.

A Native American talking circle

In the traditional ceremony, the shaman opens the ceremony by burning sage and touching each participant with an eagle feather. The objective of that ritual is to remind each person that they are in a special place and should shed whatever clings to them from the outside world. Then the leader talks about why the participants are gathered here at this time.

During the ceremony, an object is passed from hand to hand. It could be a talisman that has special significance. As the object comes around, each person is allowed to speak without time limit, but must stop as soon as the object is passed along. No one else is allowed to speak until the object comes into his or her hand.

If your family has an important issue to discuss, you might try creating your own version of this ritual. Have each participant in turn hold an object that has meaning to the family and speak while others remain silent. As the object makes the rounds of each family member, all of the aspects of the issue will gradually emerge.

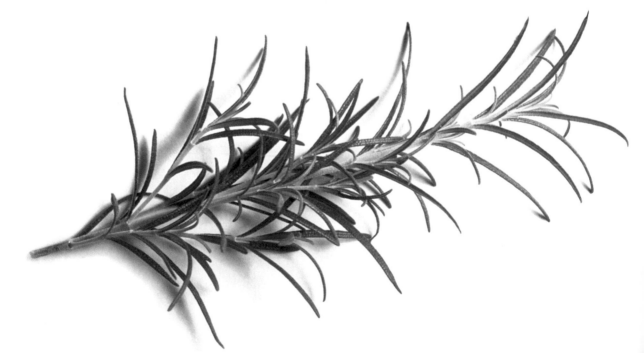

Chapter 8
Professional treatments
Options for a thorough cleanse

Only trained professionals can safely apply many of the more powerful purification techniques. You will need to go to a clinic or spa, and costs may be high. This is what you can expect from each type of treatment.

Chelation therapy

A technique that removes heavy metals, including nickel, lead, mercury, cadmium, and arsenic, from the bloodstream. Chelating agents grab onto them like a claw, bind with them, and pull them out through the urine, sweat or stool. There are several of them, and each has an affinity for different metals.

Benefits of chelation
• Gets rid of heavy-metal toxicity.
• Reduces free radical damage.
Smoking negates chelation therapy, as will large amounts of alcohol.

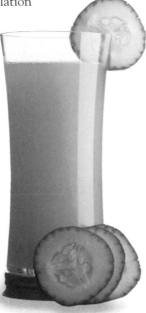

How is it done?
Patients receive an intravenous drip of vitamins, minerals and a chelating agent. Nothing is taken out of the body, and blood is not run through a machine. It can take from ½ hour to 3 hours, depending on what kind of chelating agent is used. You may need up to 30 treatments.

Chelation can lower your blood pressure or blood sugar level, so you may feel a little tired or dizzy. If this happens to you, immediately ask for some food during the chelation therapy, drink a glass of water or take a little walk.

Who does it?
To find a practitioner, check on the internet.

BETTER BOWEL HEALTH

You can't do colonic irrigation therapy on your own, but you can adjust your diet to help your bowel health.

Don't overdo binding food like pasta, bread, rice and potatoes. Eat lots of salad and drink raw vegetable juice – it's full of healthy enzymes.

Colonic irrigation

Also called colonic hydrotherapy, high colonic and colonic hydration, it involves cleaning out the large bowel with water.

It may be time for colonic hydrotherapy if you have: bloating, excessive burping, flatulence, poor digestion and stomach ache after meals.
Warning It's off-limits if you're pregnant.

Benefits of colonic irrigation
- Minimizes bloat, distension and feeling full.
- Increases energy.
- Nutrients are better absorbed.
- Parasites are removed.

How is it done?
A speculum, connected to a water feed tube and a waste tube, is inserted through the rectum. The tubing used in this process should be disposable. The goal is to get rid of the hard, black matter that cakes the walls of the colon (see pages 21 and 60). It's formed from years of additives, preservatives, processed foods and junk foods.

How long does it take?
The usual course is three treatments within ten days of each other.

Who does it?
Colonic hydrotherapists do not have to be doctors, but they should be trained by a recognized association. You can find one through the internet or ask your doctor.

Kneipp method: external hydration

The Kneipp method of purification uses the application of alternate hot and cold water and herbs to cleanse and detoxify the skin and to improve circulation to the arms and legs.

Benefits of the Kneipp method
Circulatory system, respiratory system, lymph system and digestive system improve, because they are all stimulated to contract and dilate.

How is it done?
Lavender and rosemary are used in a hot herbal bath, which is followed by a chilled bath, after which the body reacts to warm itself.

Then even more heat is applied using a herbal wrap. After that, the therapist applies cooler water and allows the person's body to dry on its own. The next step is a massage, usually a traditional Swedish massage.

Contrast baths for arms and legs can be given. The legs are warmed up to the knee in warm water, just above body temperature, then they are plunged into some cold water for a few seconds, so there's a constriction in the skin.

Then 20 minutes of rest or meditation follow.

How long does it take?
Each session of hydrotherapy will take about half an hour to complete. For the full effect, you have to do it several times over the course of two weeks.

Who does it?
Hydrotherapy of this kind is usually done by a massage therapist, with at least two years of training in physiotherapy. Ask your doctor for more information.

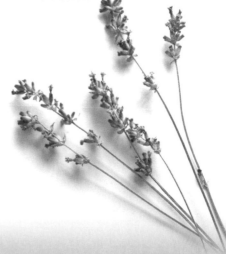

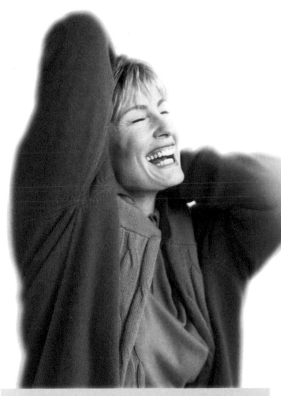

KNEIPP THERAPY IN A TUB

You can do this treatment at home, but for practical reasons, you should stick to arm and leg treatments. You need two large tubs. Showerheads don't do the job adequately. Stand with both feet in a large tub of warm water, 40°C to 41°C (104°F to 106°F) . The water should come up to your knees. Allow your legs to get good and warm. Then step into a tub of cooler water, 18°C to 21°C (64°F to 70°F) until they cool down. Step out of the cool water and allow your legs to warm themselves up. Repeat this two or three times a day over several days or even a week. Allow 30 minutes per session. Warm, chill, then walk around without drying. The herbs used can include rosemary, but you can use any herbs you like, if you want to add them to the water.

Lymphatic drainage massage

Lymph is the fluid collected between cells. The lymphatic system is like a second circulatory system, distributing fluids and nutrients throughout your body. If drainage is inadequate these fluids build up, causing swelling and discomfort. The lymph can contain significant amounts of the toxic by-product of cellular metabolism.

Benefits of lymphatic drainage massage
- Reduces cellular toxins that build up in tissue.
- Treatment for lymphedema (accumulation of excess fluids resulting in inflammation);
- Encourages post-operative healing, especially after liposuction.
- Improves the appearance of cellulite and tissue swelling due to varicose veins.
- Reduces water retention during menstruation.
- Flushes out toxins.
- Improves circulation.

How is it done?
The massage therapist uses rhythmic, nearly circular strokes to move lymphatic fluids back toward the nearest lymph node.

How long does it take?
If you're having the treatment for cellulite, swelling or water retention associated with menstruation or surgery, it'll take approximately 15 treatments to get any really noticeable results – two treatments per week over the course of a month, followed by one treatment per month to maintain results. However, for those suffering from lymphedema, the treatment may be more often. Each treatment lasts about 45 minutes.

Who does it?
Physiotherapists, trained clinicians and massage therapists can perform lymphatic drainage. Talk to your GP practice or look on the internet.

If you're not suffering from a serious medical condition but are experiencing occasional swelling, here are some techniques to try.

- Follow a low-salt diet
- Wear compression stockings
- Elevate your lower extremities
- Exercise and massage your arms and legs
- Refrain from sitting in a position with your knees flexed for a long period

Panchakarma

Ayurveda, India's ancient tradition of medicine, includes a method for body detoxification called panchakarma. It uses a number of different purification therapies that include herbal oil massage, herbal laxatives and enemas, body wraps, and herbal steam, all tailored to the individual's body type. The idea is to use these therapies to eliminate toxins from the body. Ayurvedic medicine views toxins as the root causes of disease.

Benefits of Panchakarma

- Deep relaxation and a sense of well-being.
- Elimination of fatigue.
- Enhanced digestive power.
- Faster elimination of waste products.
- Improved circulation.
- Improved strength, endurance, energy, vitality and mental clarity.
- Minimized negative influences of stress.
- Removal of toxins from body and mind.
- Smooth skin.
- Strengthened immune system.

Warning Panchakarma should not be given to pregnant or menstruating women.

How is it done?

Extreme traditional panchakarma techniques are modified for Westerners.

Before treatment, follow a diet of cooked vegetables, lentil soups and light grains. Also eat ghee early every morning, on an empty stomach. It pulls out toxins by making them soluble. They find their way to the bloodstream, the liver clears them into the bile, and finally they reach the intestine. At that point, a laxative such as castor oil is used to clean the bowel. Eat liquid foods for the rest of the day.

Once at the clinic, a vegetarian diet starts. Every day herbalized oils are rubbed onto the body. Then either a relaxation treatment or a heat treatment is given to open up the circulatory channels of the body, which increases circulation to the extremities. At the end of each treatment day an enema is given.

How long does it take?

Ideally, a course of treatment should last at least five days (not including four or five days of preparation done at home). Traditionally, panchakarma is carried out once a year.

Who does it?

Specialist clinics do the cleansing. Find your nearest one by looking on the internet.

Acupuncture-based therapies

Acupuncture, acupressure, reflexology and Shiatsu are based on the traditional Oriental view that stimulating certain points on the surface of the body with either thin-gauge, painless needles or with the fingers, hands and feet, can affect various organs and systems in the body. The points are located along 'meridians', or energy channels that run through the body and along the surface of the skin.

Acupuncture, in particular, can be helpful as a part of a general detoxification programme. It has a natural diuretic effect, so it helps to eliminate toxins through the urinary tract.

Benefits of acupuncture-based therapies

• Helps the body reach a state of balance.
• Useful for older sufferers from arthritis, osteoporosis, and general aches and pains.
• Repairs damage caused by abuse of drugs, alcohol and sex.
• Restores energy, counteracts nervousness, anxiety or depression.
• Useful for sports injuries.
• Reduces the negative effects of chemotherapy.
• Helps people to stop smoking.

How is it done?

Acupuncture uses small needles and acupressure uses the fingertips to stimulate various points. Reflexology does the same thing, but it concentrates on points located on the feet. Shiatsu adds various massage techniques, such as stretching, rolling and percussion to stimulate the trigger points in the body.

How long does it take?

Sessions last from 30 to 60 minutes. For detoxification, people stay in their programmes for six months or more. If you want to generally improve your health, then a tune-up once every few months is appropriate.

Who does it?

Acupuncture-based therapies are done by practitioners who train in the appropriate techniques. To find a good therapist, start with a recommendation from a friend, or better yet, a referral from your doctor. You could also try to find someone online.

DO-IT-YOURSELF-SHIATSU

There is a type of shiatsu called Do-in. You perform do-in by kneading the muscles of your arms, legs and abdomen the way you would knead bread, but always in a clockwise direction. You can also give yourself a reflexology treatment by pressing on the appropriate trigger points on your feet. You'll need to find a book with a chart to show you where they are.

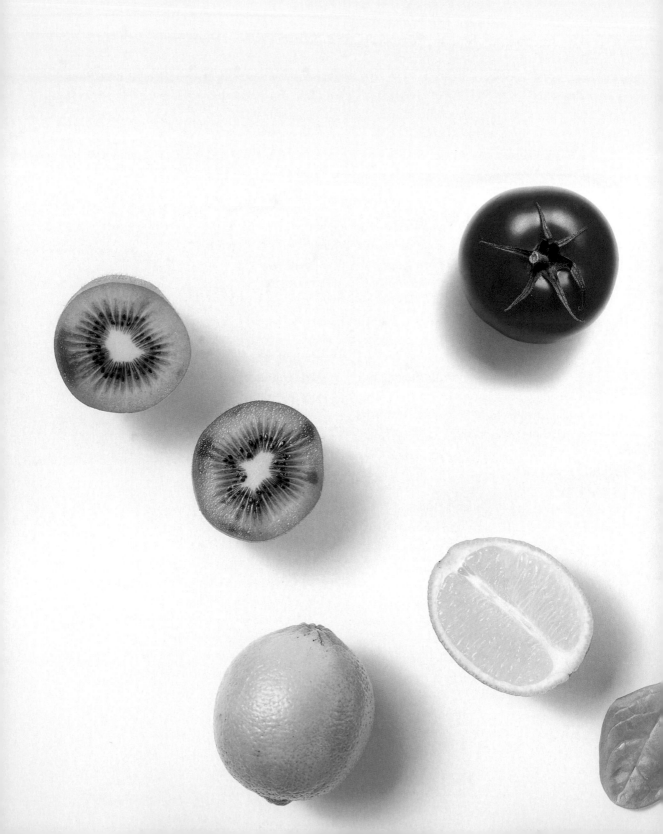

The Detox! plans
Your strategy for better health

This section guides you towards your personal
health goals. It includes the 7-day detox plan,
a general purpose purification routine, followed
by a selection of cleansing yoga exercises.
Next comes a chapter of delicious, healthy
recipes, followed by a helpful guide to setting
up your own home spa. From there, paths will
diverge into a variety of targeted plans and instant
ideas, where you'll find strategies that are more
specific to your individual health concerns.
The final chapter closes the loop on detoxification
by helping you to eliminate the main sources of
toxicity in your life for a healthy, pure lifestyle.

Chapter 9

The 7-day detox plan
A body-cleansing routine

Give your mind and body a good spring-cleaning. This simple, yet powerfully effective programme is based on a plan developed in conjunction with Dr Peter Bennett, a naturopathic physician who lives in Vancouver, Canada.

The 7-day detox plan will help you to eliminate the poisons that your body has absorbed from air, water, food and household and personal-care products, as well as 'auto-intoxicants' such as nicotine and white sugar.

It will also help you to lose weight, gain energy and increase mental clarity and well-being. You will also find out how to relieve or even eliminate conditions caused or aggravated by environmental toxins, including headaches, fatigue, indigestion, constipation and premenstrual syndrome (PMS).

Ideally, devote a week or two each year to the full routine, but if your schedule won't allow you to devote a full week to the routine, simply adapt it. For example, you can do a weekend 'mini-cleanse' whenever you feel stressed or run-down.

No matter how long you follow the programme, get as much rest, sleep and quiet as you can while you're cleansing. You may experience a few less-than-pleasant symptoms (see 'Are you having a healing crisis?' on page 17). But rest assured they're usually signs that your body is cleansing itself of toxins.

Follow this programme only if you're a healthy, normal weight or overweight adult. Don't attempt this or any cleansing regimen if:

- You have a serious health condition (such as heart disease, diabetes, cancer, a kidney or digestive disorder, or an autoimmune disease such as lupus or rheumatoid arthritis).

- You are underweight.
- You are pregnant or nursing.
- You are anorexic or bulimic.
- You are having chemotherapy.
- You have had surgery within the last two weeks.

Don't be discouraged from undertaking purification if you have any of these conditions.

It may still be possible to detoxify, and you could well benefit greatly from doing so. You just need to do so under medical supervision. Consult your doctor for advice.

About the routine

This programme has five components that will work together to cleanse your mind as well as your body. Here's an overview.

1 Diet For the next week, you'll enjoy three meals and two snacks a day, each composed largely of fresh fruits and vegetables, whole grains and plant proteins. We'll also recommend herbal teas and supplements to help your body to purify itself and build your immunity to the toxins you really can't avoid. For more herbal options, refer to Chapter 4.

2 Physical activity Each day, you'll get at least 20 minutes – preferably 40 – of gentle activity to stimulate blood circulation and lymphatic fluid.

EVERYDAY CLEANSERS

Do the following three cleansing techniques each day that you follow the programme.

1 Take a multivitamin supplement and 1,000mg of vitamin C every morning.

2 Perform alternate nostril breathing immediately after waking up, before you get out of bed.

• Sit on the side of your bed, holding your spine straight. Gently exhale all the air from your lungs.

• Press the thumb of your right hand against your right nostril, closing off the flow of air. Inhale slowly and deeply through your left nostril until your lungs are full.

• While your lungs are still full, remove your thumb from your right nostril, press your left nostril closed with your ring finger, and exhale through your right nostril.

• Inhale through the right nostril, slowly and deeply. When your lungs are full again, close your right nostril with your thumb, as before, and exhale through your left nostril.

This completes one round. Begin with 10 rounds and work your way up to 30.

3 Perform the following end-of-the-day gratitude exercise before bed.

Do a breathing exercise Gently pinch your right nostril shut and breathe for 12 inhalations and exhalations, through your left nostril only.

Remember Place your right palm on your heartbeat region and think back:

• Recall any acts of love or kindness directed toward you in the previous 72 hours.

• Relive how you felt at the time.

• Notice your feelings and allow appreciation and gratitude to form.

• Recall emotional issues that appeared within the last 72 hours, and then the last few weeks, months and years and allow your feelings of gratitude to form.

3 **Spa treatments** Each day, you'll indulge in a treatment to purify or pamper your body, such as detoxification baths, facials and other delights.

4 **Emotional cleansing** Every day this week, you'll learn a new 'mind game'. These games are designed to turn off the negative thoughts that lead to stress, anger and depression and replace them with positive thinking, which will make you feel more optimistic and in control.

5 **Stress control** Stress is just about the most toxic body state there is. As you learn new stress-reduction techniques, continue to do the ones that seem to work best for you and make it a point to do one or two of them at least once a day.

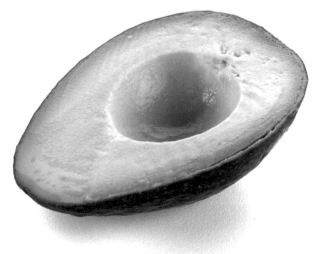

FRESH PRODUCE (ORGANIC)

Aubergine Contains nasunin, an antioxidant shown to protect cell membranes from damage.

Basil Contains compounds with antibacterial properties.

Coriander Contains volatile oils which may be antimicrobial.

Mint Aids digestion.

Parsley Contains terpenoids that may delay the onset of cancer.

Thyme Its volatile oil, thymol, increases the percentage of healthy fats in cell membranes and other cell structures.

Assorted fruits and berries Their fibre, vitamins, minerals and plant compounds support liver detoxification.

Broccoli Contains compounds that stimulate cells to produce detox enzymes.

Carrots Rich in carotenoid antioxidants that disarm free radicals.

Celery Contains coumarins that help to control free radicals.

Courgettes Contain glutathione, a sulphur-containing amino acid that is an important part of the body's antioxidant defence system.

Garlic Rich in manganese, which helps to make the antioxidant enzyme superoxide dismutase.

Green beans Good source of the trace mineral copper, needed to produce superoxide dismutase.

Lemons Good source of vitamin C.

Mushrooms Contain selenium, which plays an important role in the immune system.

Onions Contain antioxidant.

Pepper Green, red, yellow or orange. Rich source of vitamin C and beta-carotene.

Potatoes Contain chlorogenic acid, that blocks the action of cancer-causing nitrosamines in cigarette smoke.

Raisins Good source of potassium and iron.

Spring onions Contain allium, that may lower cholesterol levels and blood pressure.

Sweet potatoes or yams Contain phytochelatins, chemicals shown to bind to harmful substances such as copper, cadmium, mercury and lead.

Swiss chard Good source of vitamin C and isothiocyanates.

Tomatoes Contain lycopene, a nutrient found to protect against cancers, of the stomach, colon, mouth and oesophagus.

REFRIGERATED/FROZEN FOODS

Broccoli florets Contain B vitamins and vitamin C.

Cheese, blue, Cheddar and cottage Reduced-fat where possible.

Cheese, Gouda, smoked

Eggs Organic if possible. Rich in choline, a substance that assists with the removal of fat in the liver.

Milk Skimmed or soya.

Rice milk (optional; for protein shakes).

Shrimp or prawns Excellent source of selenium, for phase one detoxification.

Sour cream Fat-free, if possible.

Tofu Both soft and firm. Good source of the trace mineral zinc.

Yogurt Fat-free plain, containing live bacterial cultures to help to fortify the immune system.

CANNED GOODS

Cannellini beans Low salt, canned. Contain minerals and B vitamins.

Kidney beans Low salt, canned. High in fibre, to speed food through the digestive tract.

Tomato purée Canned (organic).
Tomato sauce Canned (organic if possible).
Tuna Canned in brine.
NUTS AND SEEDS
Almonds Good source of trace minerals manganese and copper.
Sunflower seeds Raw. Good source of selenium.
Walnuts Rich in the compound ellagic acid, which detoxifies potential cancer-causing substances.
GRAINS
Barley Good source of soluble fibre.
Brown rice Rich in manganese, selenium and magnesium.
Oatmeal Good source of selenium.
OILS AND FATS
Tahini Bottled. 1 tablespoon provides 12 percent of your daily requirement of copper and thiamin, a B vitamin that helps to convert food into energy.
Any one or more of the following:
Butter Organic.
Flaxseed oil High in essential fatty acids, which support liver detoxification.
Olive oil
Sunflower seed oil High in essential fatty acids. *Caution* Too much can make your body prone to inflammation.
HERBS, SPICES, AND FLAVOURINGS
Apple-cider vinegar
Balsamic vinegar
Chilli-garlic paste
Cinnamon May help to stop growth of bacteria and fungi, including candida yeast.
Cumin May stimulate the secretion of pancreatic enzymes.

Curry
Dill Its volatile oils may help to neutralize carcinogens in cigarette smoke.
Fennel seeds Aid digestion.
Ginger Fresh or dried. Its gingerols may inhibit the growth of cancer cells.
Honey Good for sore throats and removing phlegm.
Hot-pepper sauce
Minced onion
Oregano Contains thymol and rosmarinic acid with potent antioxidant properties.
Red pepper
Rice vinegar
Rosemary Contains substances that stimulate the immune system, increase circulation, and improve digestion.
Sesame oil
Soy sauce Reduced sodium.
Tumeric Reverses liver damage caused by toxins; lowers levels of cancer-causing compounds in smokers.
Pure vanilla flavouring
Worcestershire sauce
AT THE HEALTH FOOD STORE
Almond oil
Aloe vera gel
Bentonite or green clay
Chamomile tea
Essential oil of lavender, grapefruit, juniper and rosemary
Kelp powder
Lemon balm tea
Natural-bristle dry skin brush
Passionflower tea
Rice protein powder (optional)
Sea salt
Tamari

MISCELLANEOUS
Baking soda
Buffing cream
Chamois skin buffer
Epsom salts

Nail polish formulated without dibutyl phthalate (DBP) (optional).
Nail-polish remover formulated without toluene and formaldehyde (optional).
Paraffin wax (optional; for foot treatment).

Day 1

Menu

Your detoxifying tea Drink up to 3 cups or 3 tincture dosages of either dandelion leaf or buchu teas, hot or iced. These teas have a diuretic effect, helping the kidneys to eliminate toxins through the urine. **Caution** Do not drink these teas if you are taking a medication that has a diuretic effect, such as spironolactone. These teas may increase the effect of these drugs and lead to possible cardiovascular side effects. See 'Herbal detox recipes' on page 83 for preparation details and dosage information.

Breakfast Breakfast rice pudding (page 103).

Snack 1 Fruit smoothie (page 129) or any of the cleansing beverages in Chapter 4.

Lunch Salad with Sunflower seed dressing (page 127), baked potato.

Snack 2 Rice protein shake (page 128) or any of the cleansing beverages in chapter 4.

Dinner Aubergine bake with herb sauce (page 114).

Detoxercise

Take a brisk 20-minute walk, preferably in the morning. In the afternoon or evening, exercise again for 20 minutes, by walking, ballroom dancing, bicycling, skipping, swimming, yoga, aerobics or strength training. Do not work above your ability level, and stop to rest as often as you feel you need to.

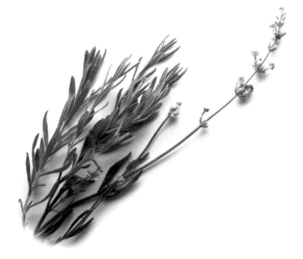

Spa care

Hot Epsom salts/lavender-oil bath followed by dry skin brushing Epsom salts, or magnesium sulphate, will help to draw toxins out of the body, including some heavy metals (mercury, lead and aluminum), car exhaust, solvents and many other modern-day toxins.

Most people are deficient in magnesium, and many of the body's detoxification pathways are dependent on it. The lavender oil promotes tranquillity. Several studies have shown that lavender has profound stress-reducing benefits.

You will need 1 cup of Epsom salts and 2–3 drops of lavender oil.

Fill your bath with water that's as hot as you can stand (to promote sweating) and add the Epsom salts and oil. Soak for up to 30 minutes. Afterwards, take a cool shower to wash toxins from the surface of your skin.

HERBAL DETOX RECIPES

You should be able to purchase most of these herbs in tea-bag form from a health food store. Follow the dosage instructions on the label. The doses provided assume that you are taking only one of these herbs at a time. Note: Talk to your doctor before adding herbal remedies to your health care regimen.

BUCHU (*Barosma betulina*)
Dosage Three doses per day.
Tea preparation Infuse 1 tsp in 1 cup of water for 10 minutes. Strain and drink.
Tincture Take ½ tsp of tincture 1:5.

CHAMOMILE (*Matricaria recutita*)
Dosage Three doses per day.
Tea preparation Infuse 1 to 4 tsp in 1 cup of water for 10 minutes. Strain and drink.
Tincture Take ¼ to 1 tsp of tincture 1:1.

DANDELION LEAF (*Taraxacum officinalis*)
Dosage Three doses per day.
Tea preparation Infuse 1 tbsp dried dandelion leaf in a cup of water for 10 minutes. Strain and drink.
Tincture Take 1 tsp of tincture 1:5 diluted in water, juice or tea.

LEMON BALM (*Melissa officinalis*)
Dosage Three doses per day.
Tea preparation Infuse 1 to 2 tsp in 1 cup of water for 10 minutes. Strain and drink.
Tincture Take ½ to 1 tsp of tincture 1:1.

PASSIONFLOWER (*Passiflora incarnata*)
Dosage Three doses per day.
Tea preparation Infuse 1 tsp in 1 cup of water for 10 minutes. Strain and drink.
Tincture Take ½ tsp of tincture 1:5.

UVA URSI (*Arctostaphyllos uva-ursi*)
Dosage Three doses per day.
Tea preparation Infuse 1 tsp in 1 cup of water for 10 minutes. Strain and drink.
Tincture Take 1 tsp of tincture 1:5.

YARROW (*Achillea millefolium*)
Dosage Three doses per day.
Tea preparation Infuse 1 to 2 tsp in 1 cup of water for 10 minutes. Strain and drink.
Tincture Take ½ to 1 tsp of tincture 1:1.

Dry skin brushing In this technique, you brush your whole body with a soft, natural bristle brush (available in health stores) to stimulate the circulation of blood and lymphatic fluid.

Using short, brisk strokes, brush each body part in the order that follows, and always brush towards your heart. Do not wet the brush, and do not allow anyone else to use it. As with all these techniques, the highest standards of hygiene are essential.

- The fronts and backs of your arms, moving from your fingertips up into your armpits.
- Each leg, front and back, starting at your feet and brushing upwards.
- The bottoms of your feet.
- Your buttocks, abdomen and lower back.
- Your chest and upper back.
- With a dry washcloth (not a brush) brush your face with downward strokes.

Mind game

A forgiveness exercise Forgiving those who have wronged you – or forgiving yourself – may help you to purge emotional toxins such as sadness and anger. Try this exercise to help yourself to feel forgiveness towards others and yourself.

Sit in a quiet, comfortable place. Close your eyes and imagine that there is a circle of light around you. Ask yourself 'Who have I not forgiven?' Wait for someone's face to appear in your mind's eye. Invite this person into your circle. Visualize looking into his or her eyes and complete one or both of the following sentences:

'What I learned from you is …'

'You taught me …'

When you've finished, thank that person. If you wish, you may repeat the exercise, continuing to thank him or her until you feel at peace. Then say:

'I forgive you. I release you. Go in peace.'

Say goodbye. And with love, watch him or her leave your circle and disappear. Repeat this exercise as often as you need to with as many people as you need to.

Stress-reduction technique

Soak in a sound bath To take a 'sound bath', put some relaxing music on your stereo and lie in a comfortable position on a sofa or on the floor near the speakers. For a deeper experience, you can wear headphones to focus your attention and to avoid being distracted by others. Allow the music to wash over you, sweeping away the day's stress. Focus on your breathing, letting it deepen, slow and become regular.

Day 2

Menu

Your detoxifying tea Drink up to 4 cups of the same teas you enjoyed on day 1. (See caution in day 1.)

Breakfast Fresh fruit salad with almonds (page 122).

Snack 1 Fruit smoothie (page 129) or any of the cleansing beverages in chapter 4.

Lunch Salad with Tomato & dill dressing (page 127), Minestrone soup (page 116).

Snack 2 Rice protein shake (page 128) or any of the cleansing beverages in chapter 4.

Dinner Very vegetable omelette (page 113).

Detoxercise

Take a brisk 20-minute walk, preferably in the morning. In the afternoon or evening, do another 20-minute session of one of the activities listed under Day 1 Detoxercise on page 82. Also, do the 'Cardio with a kick' programme on page 94.

Spa care

Sea salt and baking soda bath, followed by sea salt body scrub Along with sea salt, baking soda helps to relax the body and may also eliminate trace toxins that your body has been exposed to in your workplace.

You will need 1 cup baking soda, 1 cup sea salt and 1 or 2 drops essential oil of your choice

Fill your tub with the hottest water you can stand (to promote sweating) and add the baking soda, sea salt and oil. Soak for up to 30 minutes. Afterward, take a cool shower to wash toxins from the surface of your skin.

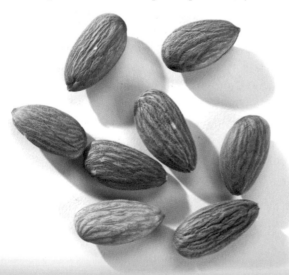

Enjoy this fragrant scrub after you've completed today's hydrotherapy treatment.

You will need 1 cup fine sea salt, ½ cup almond oil and 10 drops each of grapefruit and juniper essential oils.

Combine all the ingredients in a small bowl and blend thoroughly. Standing in the bathtub, spread the mixture onto your damp skin and massage in with gentle circular motions. Shower off the mixture, using water as cold as you can stand.

Mind game

Autogenic training Autogenics, which means 'self-generation', is designed to generate deep relaxation in a practical way. Proponents of autogenic training believe that it stimulates bloodflow and deep relaxation. The idea is to get yourself comfortable and give your body a series of instructions.

To begin, sit or lie in a comfortable position. Close your eyes and take a few deep breaths. As you exhale, repeat the following to yourself:

- My hands and arms are warm and heavy. (5 times)
- My feet and legs are warm and heavy. (5 times)
- My abdomen is calm and comfortable. (5 times)
- My breathing is deep and even. (10 times)
- My heartbeat is regular. (10 times)
- My forehead is cool. (5 times)
- When I open my eyes, I will remain relaxed and refreshed. (3 times)

Take a moment to move your hands, arms, legs and feet around a bit. Rotate your head, open your eyes and, if you're lying down, sit up.

While doing this exercise, note what is happening to your body, but don't consciously try to analyze it. If your mind wanders, simply bring it back to your instructions. Do the exercise for 2 minutes at least once a day.

Stress-reduction technique

Shavasana Yoga pose The Shavasana pose is also known as the Corpse pose, because you're simply lying on your back with your eyes closed. In reality, however, you'll emerge from this pose (which takes only 5 minutes) feeling more refreshed and alive. Do Shavasana twice a day all week – once after you perform your daily Detoxercise, and again right before bed.

Lie on your bed on your back, and spread your feet about 45cm (18in) apart. Place your hands, palms up, about 15cm (6in) from your sides. Ease yourself into the pose, making sure your body is symmetrical. Let your thighs, knees and toes relax and turn gently outward. Close your eyes and breathe deeply and slowly from your abdomen. Feel your weight pulling you deeper into relaxation. Sink deeper with each exhalation, allowing your hands, feet, abdomen, throat and eyes to get heavier and heavier. Repeat for 50 deep, relaxing, cleansing breaths.

Day 3

Menu

Your detoxifying tea Drink up to 3 cups of either yarrow or chamomile tea. These herbs are diaphoretic, meaning that they increase elimination of toxins through sweating. See 'Herbal detox recipes' on page 83 for preparation details and dosage information.

Breakfast Fruit melba breakfast sundae (page 104).

Snack 1 Fresh fruit salad with almonds (page 122).

Lunch Salad with Tahini dressing (page 126); rice or baked potato.

Snack 2 Minestrone soup (page 116) or any of the cleansing beverages in Chapter 4.

Dinner Mexican red rice & beans (page 106). Save the remaining serving for tomorrow's lunch. It keeps well in the fridge.

Detoxercise

Take a brisk 20-minute walk, preferably in the morning. In the afternoon or evening, take another 20-minute walk, or do one of the activities listed under Day 1 Detoxercise on page 82. Do not work above your ability level, and stop and rest as often as you need to.

Spa Care

A 30-minute facial

1 Cleanse gently but thoroughly In a blender, combine ½ cup of oatmeal, ¾ cup of hot water, and 1 tablespoon of olive oil. Let the mixture sit until the oatmeal has absorbed much of the water. In the meantime, apply a warm, damp washcloth to your face; the warmth will open your pores. Keep the washcloth on your face until it cools, then repeat the process. (Do not scrub your face with the cloth.) Apply the cleanser, and gently rub it into your skin, making small circles with your fingertips. Rinse well with lukewarm water for at least 30 seconds. Pat your face dry with a clean, dry towel or washcloth.

2 Apply a herbal compress Mix 5 to 10 drops of lavender oil with 1 teaspoon of vinegar. Add this mixture to a quart of cool or lukewarm water. Place another clean washcloth in the warm water, wring it out, and apply the cloth to your face. Hold the washcloth to your face for 5 to 10 seconds, rinse the cloth, and repeat the process. Repeat three more times. Pat your face dry with a clean, dry towel or washcloth.

3 Steam away impurities Bring a large pot of water to a boil. Place 3 tablespoons of dried chamomile or rosemary in an old stocking or cheesecloth. Remove the boiling water from the burner and add the herbs. Let them steep for 10 minutes. Pour the hot water into a large bowl on a nonslip surface. Lean over the bowl and drape a towel over your head so that the steam rises to your face. (Keep your face at least 30cm (12in) away from the top of the pot.) Steam for 10 minutes, being careful not to scald your skin.
Note If you have blemished or sensitive skin, steam for only 5 minutes.

4 Slip into a seaweed detoxifying mask Mix 2 tablespoons of kelp powder (available at health food stores) and ¼ cup of aloe vera gel in a small bowl. Add water until the mixture is thick and smooth. Apply to your face. Relax for 10 to 20 minutes. Rinse.

5 Tone and rebalance your skin Mix 2 tablespoons of apple cider vinegar in 1 cup of water (preferably distilled water). Apply to your face with cotton balls, avoiding your eyes.

6 Replenish moisture Apply a very thin coating of olive, sunflower or flax oil to your skin. If you have oily or acne-prone skin, omit this step.

Mind game

Anger detoxification game This exercise is a lesson in deflating the power of anger. Try it even if you're not angry, and see if it doesn't help the next time your blood is boiling.

Thinking aloud, describe a situation in your life that makes you really angry. It can be a situation from the past or present. As you speak, consciously try to really whip yourself into a frenzy about it.

Stop! Think about whether this situation is worthy of such anger. Do you really need this kind of toxic emotion in your heart, threatening your physical and mental well-being?

Now, 'talk' about the same problem, using only the words 'blah, blah, blah'. Think the anger words, but say only 'blah'. Chances are, you'll start to laugh. Right now, you have just relieved yourself of a small part of the toxic burden anger places on you.

Stress-reduction technique

Calming visualizations In visualization, which is also called guided imagery, you create relaxing images to calm your mind and body by controlling your breathing and visualizing a soothing image.

Read through the following visualization once or twice before you begin this exercise. It's not important that you follow the images to the letter, just that you understand the basic premise. Let your imagination soar and create the most soothing scenario for you.

Either sit or lie in a comfortable position and close your eyes. Now, see yourself sailing high in the sky in a large, translucent bubble. You are floating above an expanse of breathtakingly beautiful countryside. Peer out from your bubble and take in your surroundings. What do you see? A little farmhouse next to a field of corn? A patch of pine trees surrounding a crystal-clear lake? Whatever you see, try to create as vivid a 'mind picture' as you can.

Now, 'land' your bubble. Step out and begin to walk. Soon, you come to a beautiful rushing waterfall. At the bottom of the waterfall, there is a deep pool of water. Step into the water. Stay there for a while and you will begin to feel all of the stress in your body leave.

Allow yourself to relax. Spend some time in this tranquility. When you are ready, step out of the water, walk back to your bubble, step in, and sail off again into the sky, calm and refreshed.

Day 4

Menu

Your detoxifying tea Drink up to 3 cups of the same teas you enjoyed on day 3.

Breakfast Berry morning crush (page 103).

Snack 1 Raw vegetables with Garlic-herb dip (page 125) or Fruit smoothie (page 129) or any of the cleansing beverages in Chapter 4.

Lunch Mexican red rice & beans (page 106) left over from last night.

Snack 2 Rice protein shake (page 128) or any of the cleansing beverages in Chapter 4.

Dinner Moroccan carrot salad with toasted cumin (page 124).

Detoxercise

Take a brisk 20-minute walk, preferably in the morning. In the afternoon or evening, take another 20-minute walk. Do not stress yourself, and stop to rest as often as you need to.

Spa care

Hand massage followed by manicure Give yourself a relaxing treatment using a detoxifying essential oil, such as lavender or rosemary. It's so easy to overlook how soothing it can be.

Hand massage

1 Place 5 drops of lavender essential oil into the palm of one hand. If using rosemary essential oil, combine 10 drops of the oil with 1 teaspoon of almond oil and place in the palm of one hand. Rub your palms together until you feel heat.

2 Squeeze the fleshy part of your right hand between your left thumb and forefinger, with your thumb on the top side, for 10 seconds.

3 Massage your entire right palm with your left thumb. Start from the outside of your palm, working in a circular motion to the inside. For deeper treatment, search out sore spots, press with the thumb, and hold for 10 seconds.

4 Massage your left hand in the same way.

Manicure

Note Before you begin, sterilize your file with rubbing alcohol or peroxide to avoid transferring bacteria from a previous manicure to your nails.

1 Remove old nail polish, then, using an emery board, file your nails.

2 Soak your cuticles in lukewarm to warm soapy water for 5 minutes to soften them.

3 Use an orange wood stick to push back your cuticles. Do not to cut your cuticles, which can cause infection and damage your nails.

4 Apply a small amount of buffing cream to your nails and buff in one direction across each nail, using a natural chamois skin buffer. Rinse and dry your nails.

If you use polish

5 Apply a base coat, which keeps your nails from discolouring and allows coloured polish to go on more smoothly.

6 Allow the base coat to dry for at least 15 minutes. Then apply the first coat of colour polish. Wait 5 minutes, then apply a second coat.

7 Apply a protective topcoat and let it dry.

Note To keep this spa treatment toxin-free, select nail polish removers formulated without the toxic chemicals toluene and formaldehyde. Also, avoid nail polish that contains the chemical dibutyl phthalate (DBP).

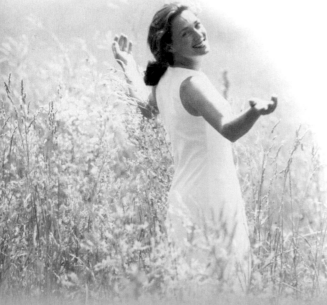

Mind game

Surrender to tranquility To purify yourself of toxic emotions, you need to learn to let them go. This simple but powerful exercise, which uses one blank sheet of standard-size paper, can help you do just that.

Think of a problem, big or small, that has been worrying you. Write it on the paper. Really focus on its negativity; state exactly how it's causing anxiety in your life and disturbing your tranquility. Write as much as you wish.

1 Fold your paper into a paper plane. Count to three, and as you reach three, sail your plane – and your worry – into the air with a cheer or a whoop. If you don't know how to make a paper plane, then place the paper in a deep bowl and set it on fire. As you watch it burn, cheer or whoop.

2 Close your eyes and give a soft sigh of satisfaction. Repeat the sigh three times, increasing the volume until your whole body gets into the act.

Stress-reduction technique

Circle breathing Circle breathing is a way to relax and calm the mind and body. Whenever you feel stressed, remember that you have a choice to practice stress or to practice peace. Then take 5 to 10 'circle breaths'. Try to perform this exercise at least five times today.

1 Begin your breaths Inhale and stretch your arms over your head, then give a sigh of relief and lower your arms as you exhale.

2 Bring in the peace Now imagine that you're inhaling a stream of peaceful energy into a spot just below your navel.

3 Move it on up Inhale the warm stream into the base of your spine, then imagine it travelling up your back to the top of your head.

4 Complete the circle Now exhale, and mentally follow your 'out' breath down the front of your body to the point below your navel where you'll begin your next 'in' breath. Your breath has now

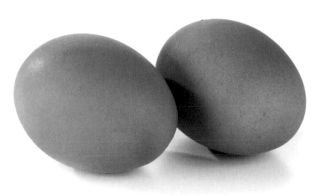

made a full circle up the back of your body, down the front, and back to the starting place just below your navel.

5 *Maintain a gentle focus* Continue this breathing pattern for 5 to 10 breaths.

Day 5

Menu

Your detoxifying tea Drink up to 3 cups of lemon balm, chamomile or passionflower teas. These teas have a sedative effect, helping to promote calmness and tranquility. See 'Herbal detox recipes' on page 83.

Breakfast Very vegetable omelette (page 113).

Snack 1 Fruit smoothie (page 129) or any of the cleansing beverages in Chapter 4.

Lunch Barley salad with smoked cheese (page 120); save the remaining serving for tomorrow's lunch.

Snack 2 Rice protein shake (see page 128) or any of the cleansing beverages in Chapter 4.

Dinner Roasted vegetable salad with balsamic & basil vinaigrette (see page 121).

Detoxercise

Don't take a walk today unless you really want to. It's good to rest your body, but you can do one of the activities listed under Day 1 Detoxercise on page 82 for 20 minutes. Do not work above your ability level, and stop to rest when you need to.

Spa care

Soothing scalp massage, followed by yogurt hair mask This simple treatment melts away tension and also improves the health and appearance of your hair by bringing fresh blood and nutrients to your hair follicles. Sitting in a comfortable chair, gently massage your scalp for 10 minutes, spreading your fingers wide and moving your fingertips in a circular motion across your scalp.

Follow with the yogurt hair mask, which is recommended for all hair types.

You will need 1 whole egg plus 1 egg yolk and 225ml (8 fl oz) natural yogurt (not fat-free).

Put a clean towel on a radiator or in a tumble dryer to warm up. Beat together the egg and yogurt. Coat your freshly shampooed hair with the mixture, and pile your hair on top of your head. Wrap your hair in the warm towel. Ease into a steamy bath and relax. After 20 minutes, drain the bath, remove the towel, and take a cool shower to rinse the mixture out of your hair. It's important to use cool water because water that's too hot will cook the egg and make it difficult to remove.

Mind game

Think yourself tranquil Virtually every second that you're conscious, you are listening to a silent interior dialogue with yourself that provides a running commentary about your life, feelings and problems, as well as the world itself. It also has a powerful effect on your feelings, beliefs and attitudes, and reinforces how you see yourself.

Affirmations are positive, powerful statements used to boost self-esteem and confidence. As you repeat the affirmations over and over, your subconscious mind comes to believe them and replaces that negative interior dialogue with a more positive one. Emil Coué, a French psychotherapist who practiced in the early 20th century, made perhaps the most famous affirmation 'Every day, in every way, I am getting better and better'.

Affirmations are worded in a positive rather than negative way, and they are grounded in the present rather than the future.

Try to come up with five affirmations that will replace the negative inner dialogue in your head. Here are some examples.

- My good thoughts and good actions produce good results.
- I am blessed with right thoughts and good actions.
- I let go of the past.
- I say yes to life.

Stress-reduction technique

Write your heart out Keeping a diary is a valuable way to release your most private thoughts and feelings. While it might seem time-consuming, setting aside just 10 to 15 minutes to put your thoughts into words may help to soothe your stress and its physical symptoms. As a bonus, writing about your feelings can help you to increase your self-knowledge, nurture your spirituality and tap into your unconscious mind.

Set aside 10 to 15 minutes and just write whatever comes into your head. Do not write at your computer. Your feelings will flow more naturally when you use a pen or pencil and a pad of paper. There's no rule about how much or how often to write. Just one paragraph a day is fine, and you don't have to write a detailed report of your day. You might want to focus on one particular person, event or problem and write about that.

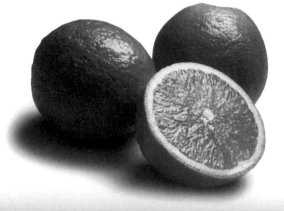

Day 6

Menu

Your detoxifying tea Drink up to 3 cups of the same teas you enjoyed on day 5.

Breakfast Select any of the breakfasts from days 1 to 5.

Snack 1 Fruit smoothie (page 129) or any of the cleansing beverages in chapter 4.

Lunch Barley salad with smoked cheese (page 120), left over from yesterday.

Snack 2 Rice protein shake (page 128) or any of the cleansing beverages in chapter 4.

Dinner Indian-spiced potatoes & spinach (page 119) - save half for tomorrow's lunch.

Detoxercise

Take a brisk 20-minute walk, preferably in the morning. In the afternoon or evening, take a second 20-minute walk. Don't do any exercises today; just give your body a rest.

Spa care

Paraffin foot dip and pedicure Your feet work hard for you – now's their time to get the royal treatment. This treatment will leave your feet looking and feeling soft and silky smooth.

Paraffin foot dip (optional) Melt paraffin wax in an old pot or saucepan that you will use just for this purpose. Massage 1 tablespoon of olive oil into each foot. When the wax is slightly cool to the touch, dip each foot into the wax four or five times. Wrap each foot in a plastic bag. Relax for about 15 minutes.

The paraffin will harden into a waxy foot 'mask'. Remove the plastic bags, then peel off the wax. Your feet will be silky-smooth for about two weeks.

Pedicure

1 Remove old polish Add a few drops of your favourite essential oil to warm water and soak your feet for 10 minutes. When you have finished soaking, rinse your feet with cold water, dry them and buff away calluses and dead skin with a pumice stone or foot file.

2 Trim your nails straight across using a pair of straight-edged clippers. Use an emery board to file your nails.

3 Soak your cuticles in lukewarm to warm soapy water for 5 minutes to soften them.

4 Use an orange wood stick to push back your cuticles. Do not to cut your cuticles, which can cause infection and damage your nails.

If you apply polish

5 Twist a tissue and weave it between your toes to keep them separate. Then apply polish and let it dry for at least 30 minutes.

If you don't use polish

6 Apply a liberal dollop of a thick moisturizing cream Then slip on a pair of big, fluffy socks to retain the moisture.

Mind game

Giving negative thoughts a makeover If you believe in the power of positive thinking, then you'll probably benefit from this exercise in rational-emotive behaviour therapy (REBT). This maintains that to a large extent we don't get upset by things or events, but by the view we take of them. When we replace irrational, self-defeating beliefs with rational ones, we are happier and more productive.

The following exercise can help you to ferret out the irrational beliefs that may be causing you worry and stress and replace them with rational beliefs. You'll be amazed at how much stress relief is packed into this simple technique.

Pick your topic On a piece of paper, write down a description of an event that provoked a specific negative emotion, such as fear or depression.

Describe your negative feeling In one sentence, write down your number one anxious thought about this event.

Balance it out In one sentence, write down a short, clear and rational statement to counter the negative thought above.

Stress-reduction technique

Be mindful Like our bodies, our minds are constantly going, going, going. Most of us are constantly either planning the future or lamenting the past. The happy medium is to be 'mindful', which is to have a heightened awareness of the present. Mindfulness may not only diminish stress, anxiety and depression, but may also transform a person's actual approach to life itself.

Mindfulness-based stress reduction (MBSR) is a meditation technique with proven benefits in the reduction of stress symptoms. Formal practice of MBSR involves true meditation. But informally, you can practice mindfulness in the most ordinary activities, even brushing your teeth or washing the dishes. The exercise below can help you to experience mindfulness. To do this exercise, you'll need an orange.

Take a few deep breaths and relax your body. Now, tune everything out except for this orange in your hand. Turn it this way and that, absorbing its orangeness. Examine its texture and shape, and notice how it feels in your hand. Smell it. Don't make a judgment about this orange; simply see it. Let go of any ideas of how this exercise will help you; just be accepting and aware of each passing moment. Take a moment to appreciate where the orange came from. Notice the wonderful smell as you begin to peel it. Now eat the orange slowly, noting the taste and texture of every bite. Follow each bite with your attention as you slowly chew and swallow it. Now, take this nonjudgmental, accepting, observant attitude and apply it to your daily life.

Day 7

Menu

Your detoxifying tea Drink up to 3 cups of the same teas you enjoyed on day 5.

Breakfast Select any of the breakfasts from days 1 to 5 or try Apple pancakes (page 102).

Snack 1 Fruit smoothie (page 129) or any of the cleansing beverages in Chapter 4.

Lunch Indian-spiced potatoes & spinach (page 119), left over from yesterday.

Snack 2 Rice protein shake (page 128) or any of the cleansing beverages in Chapter 4.

Dinner Barley with ginger & broccoli (page 107).

Detoxercise

Take a brisk 20-minute walk, preferably in the morning. In the afternoon or evening, take a second 20-minute walk and do the 'Cardio with a kick' programme on page 94. Do not work above your ability level, and rest as often as you need to.

Spa care

The scented clay body wrap A body wrap eliminates toxins, calms your mind and revitalizes your skin. Today, virtually every high-priced spa offers wraps featuring detoxifying ingredients such as muds, seaweeds and herbs.

A do-it-yourself body wrap requires only a few simple tools – an old cotton sheet to wrap yourself in, three towels, a pillow or cushion for your neck and an inexpensive foil thermal blanket to keep you warm. Drink lots of water before and after your wrap to help to flush out toxins.

You will need 2 cups water, ¼ cup sea salt, 1 cup bentonite or green clay (available at health food stores), 2 tablespoons olive oil and 1 tablespoon essential oil.

1 Begin by preparing the sheet Heat a large pot of water on the stove until it's comfortably hot, but not boiling. Add the cotton sheet, stir until entirely saturated, wring it out carefully, and place it in a plastic bag. Set it aside.

2 Make the clay wrap Boil the water in a large saucepan, add the sea salt and stir until the salt is fully dissolved. Add the clay, olive oil and essential oil, and stir again. Add more water if you need to so the mixture has the consistency of a wet paste.

3 Head to the bathroom with the the clay, the sheet (still warm in the plastic bag), three towels, pillow and thermal blanket.

4 Take a warm shower to open your pores and fill the air with steam. Towel off slightly and wrap your hair in a towel. Place a dry towel on the bottom of the tub. Standing on an old towel, apply the clay mixture to your still-damp skin (excluding your face). Wrap yourself from ankles to chin in the warm, damp cotton sheet. Climb into the tub and lie on the towel, arranging the pillow to support your head and neck. Cover yourself with the thermal blanket. You may need the help of a friend or partner with this treatment.

5 Allow the clay to stay on your skin for 15 minutes or until the sheet cools. Unwrap and rinse in lukewarm water. When you're dry, follow with a dry skin brushing (page 83).

Mind game

Review of the week's techniques Pick one or two of the mind games that you found to be most effective for you. Practice these mind games again for a few minutes off and on throughout the day, with the goal of integrating them into your everyday life after you complete the programme.

Stress-reduction technique

20-minute nature walk Exposure to nature has been shown to decrease heart rate, blood pressure and other indicators of stress. As you walk, be aware of the sights, sounds and even smells of the natural world around you. Chances are, you'll go home feeling more tranquil and grounded.

Chapter 10
Detoxercise
A body-toning routine

Just as there are more ways than one for toxins to infiltrate your system, so there are more ways than one to get rid of them. Exercise – especially regular exercise – is one of the most effective.

Most experts agree that the best results come from doing not just one form of exercise – although even that is better than nothing – a combination of different types of activity will give the best all-round results.

Health professionals will walk, jog, play fast-moving games, swim and lift weights. Not only does it give an excellent all-round work-out to all the muscles, but it also stops boredom setting in.

Physical activity should be fun and interesting. The body responds best if you present it with different types of stimulation that challenge its muscles in different ways.

The best exercise detoxification routine blends the right dose of fat-burning aerobic exercise, muscle-toning strength training and range-of-motion enhancing stretching. By performing a variety of types of exercise, you ensure that your detoxification efforts are well balanced and that you cover every body region.

The 7-day plan overleaf should be followed, along with the other activities already detailed in the 7-day detox plan. It includes 30 minutes of activity a day, but add more cardio (heart-pumping aerobic) activities like walking, cycling and swimming, if you like. Bouncing on a mini-trampoline is an excellent cardiovascular and detoxifying workout. You also can do more yoga or other flexibility and balance exercises.

It's best to limit strength training to two or three days a week, however, so your muscles have a chance to rest and rebuild between sessions. You can break down your 30-minute exercise session into two 15-minute or three 10-minute chunks.

Remember, though, that exercise that is too strenuous can do more harm than good, so ease into things gently, and never continue if you start to feel ill or uncomfortable. If you have any doubts about the safety of your undertaking these exercises, discuss your plans with your doctor first.

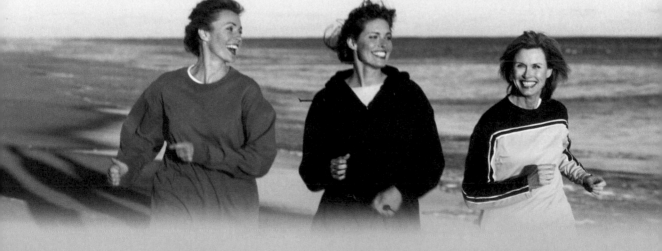

THE 7-DAY PLAN

Follow the suggestions here each day of your 7-day programme. Don't force yourself to continue if you feel it's too much for you.

Day 1	Day 2	Day 3	Day 4
• Gentle cardio of your choice (walking, cycling, swimming) for 25 minutes • Cleansing yoga series (opposite)	• Warm up with gentle cardio for 5 minutes • Detox tone-up plan (page 97) • Cool down for 5 minutes • Cardio with a kick (below)	• Warm up with gentle cardio for 5 minutes • Detox tone-up plan (page 97) • Cool down for 5 minutes	• Gentle cardio of your choice (walking, bicycling, swimming) for 25 minutes

Day 5	Day 6	Day 7
• Cleansing yoga series (opposite)	• Rest	• Cardio with a kick (below)

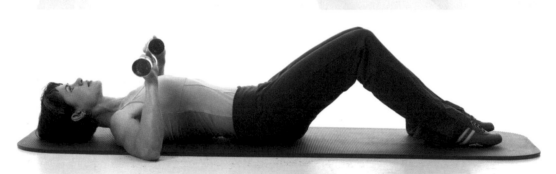

Cardio with a kick

In addition to the walking recommendations in the 7-day detox plan, here's how to boost your exercise effort in a safe and controlled way.

This programme introduces light speed work into your usual aerobic (cardio) routine. Though it specifies walking, you can do the same thing on an exercise bicycle or even in a pool, if you feel like a change of scenery, or the weather is inclement. Simply increase your effort to the specified intensity for the prescribed duration.

The number in brackets indicates the intensity on a scale of 1 to 10, with 1 being the absolute easiest (almost snoozing) and 10 being the most intense (full-out effort). This whole routine should take you about half an hour:

• Begin with an easy walking pace (3): 4 minutes
• Increase tempo to a brisk pace (6): 5 minutes
• Walk as if you're trying to catch a bus (7): 10 minutes
• Walk as fast as your feet will carry you (9): 3 minutes
• Reduce your pace to a brisk walk (6): 5 minutes
• Cool down at an easy pace (3): 3 minutes

Cleansing yoga series

Perform each position twice, moving slowly and deliberately, stretching into position only until you feel a comfortable stretch. Hold at that point for 30 seconds. Return to your starting position, rest for a few seconds, and repeat.

Downward facing dog

Benefits Reduces stress, relieves constipation and indigestion, cleanses sinuses and lungs.

A Position yourself on the floor on your hands and knees, feet flexed, toes to the floor.

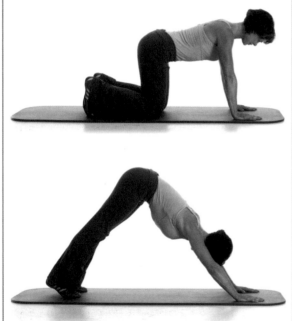

B Now press your hands and feet into the floor, raising your hips toward the ceiling. In the final position, your body should look like an upside-down V. Keep your back and legs straight, and keep lifting your coccyx toward the ceiling as you lower your heels to the floor as far as is comfortably possible.
Note This can be difficult if you are overweight or have wrist problems.

If you have trouble performing the full position, try keeping your knees slightly bent, or place your hands on something slightly higher than the floor, like an aerobic step or the first step of a staircase.

Triangle

Benefits Helps to detoxify GI tract.

A Stand with your legs wide apart, right toes pointing forward and left toes pointing out to the left. Extend your arms out to the sides, parallel with the floor.

B Slowly bend down sideways to the left as far as you can without letting yourself bend either forwards or backwards. As you do this, run your left hand along your left leg and down your left shin as far as you can, while reaching toward the ceiling with your right hand. You're aiming to ultimately get your right arm perpendicular to the floor and your left fingertips touching the floor. Once you've reached your maximum stretch, turn your head to look up toward the ceiling, and hold. Return to your starting position and repeat to the opposite side, repositioning your feet before you start.

Child's pose

Benefits Stretches spine and improves circulation.

A Kneel with the tops of your feet on the floor, toes pointed behind you. Sit back on your heels.

B Slowly lower your chest to your thighs as you stretch your arms overhead and rest your palms and forehead on the floor (or as close to it as is comfortable). If you are overweight, you can spread your legs to make space for your abdomen. Hold.

Warrior

Benefits Tones bladder, improves digestion.

A Stand tall with your feet about hip-width apart.

B Take a giant step forward with your left foot, bending that knee. Make sure your left knee does not jut out over your toes. Your left shin should be perpendicular to the floor. Turn your right foot out to the side, keeping your heel in the same place. Raise your arms over your head, palms facing each other, lifting your chin slightly. Hold, return to your starting position, and repeat, beginning with a giant step with your right foot this time.

Detox tone-up plan

Perform two sets of 10 to 12 repetitions of each exercise. Use dumbbells that are heavy enough to make the final one or two repetitions challenging.

Dumbbell squats

A Stand with your back to a chair and your feet about shoulder-width apart. Hold dumbbells up at your shoulders, palms facing in.

B Keeping your back straight, bend from your knees and hips as though you are sitting down. Don't let your knees move forward over your toes. Stop just short of touching the chair, then stand up again.

Step up

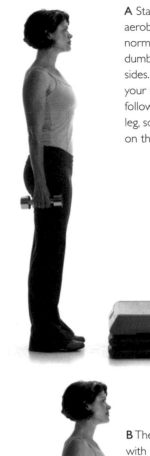

A Stand facing an aerobic step or normal step holding dumbbells at your sides. Step up with your right leg, followed by your left leg, so both feet are on the step.

B Then, step down with your right foot, followed by your left. Repeat, alternating legs, to perform a full set with each leg.

Side to sides

A Hold dumbbells at your shoulders with your palms facing in. Stand with feet wide apart, toes pointed out.

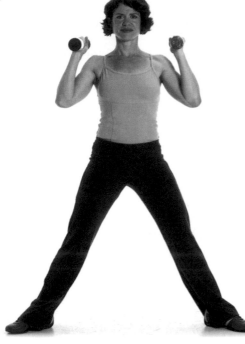

B Bend your left knee down until your left thigh is nearly parallel with the floor and your right leg is extended. Straighten back up. Then bend your right knee. Repeat, alternating legs to perform a full set with each leg.

Back fly

A Sit in a chair with your feet flat on the floor and about hip-width apart. Hold a dumbbell in each hand so the weights are at about chest level and are 30cm (12in) from your body, palms facing each other and elbows slightly bent, as if you were holding a beach ball. Bend slightly forward from your hips, about 7cm to 10cm (3in to 4in).

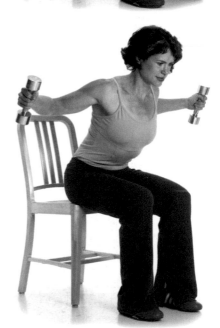

B Keeping your back straight, squeeze your shoulder blades together and pull your elbows back as far as is comfortable. Pause, then return to start.

Chest press

A Lie on the floor (or a bench, if one is available) and hold dumbbells end to end just above your chest; your elbows should be pointing out.

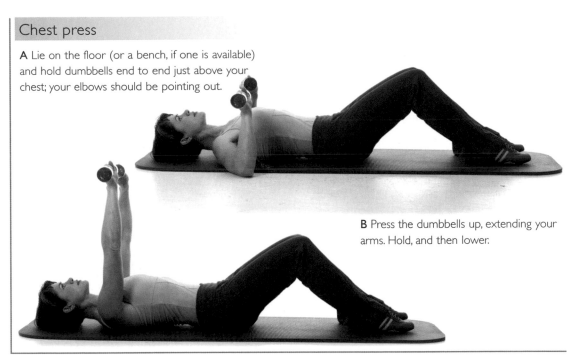

B Press the dumbbells up, extending your arms. Hold, and then lower.

Curl & press

B Slowly bend your elbows and curl the weights up toward your shoulders.

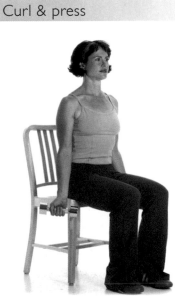

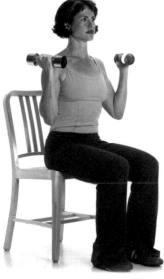

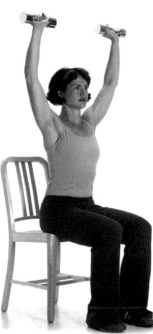

A Sit on a supportive chair (preferably one without arms), feet flat on the floor and about shoulder-width apart. Hold a dumbbell in each hand, arms extended down to your sides and palms facing out.

C Without stopping, rotate your wrists so your palms are facing forward and press the weights overhead. Pause. Slowly reverse the move back to the starting position.

Calf raise

A Stand with your legs about hip-width apart and hold dumbbells at your sides, palms facing in.

B Slowly rise up onto the balls of your feet while keeping your torso and legs straight. Hold, and then lower.

Standing crossover

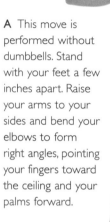

A This move is performed without dumbbells. Stand with your feet a few inches apart. Raise your arms to your sides and bend your elbows to form right angles, pointing your fingers toward the ceiling and your palms forward.

B Now contract your abdominal muscles and pull your right knee and left elbow toward one another. Pause, and return to start. Complete a set, and then switch sides.

Reverse curl

A Lie on your back with your arms extended alongside your thighs. Bend your hips and knees so your legs are over your midsection and relaxed.

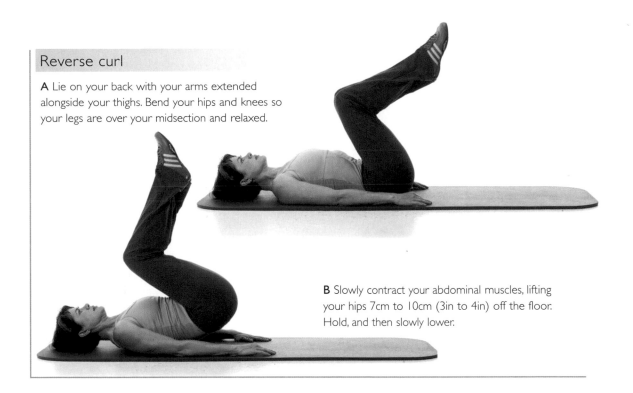

B Slowly contract your abdominal muscles, lifting your hips 7cm to 10cm (3in to 4in) off the floor. Hold, and then slowly lower.

Roll like a ball

A Sit on the floor and hug your knees to your chest. Balance on your coccyx and lift your feet, pointing your toes down towards the floor.

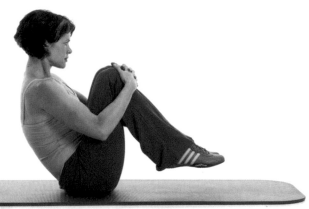

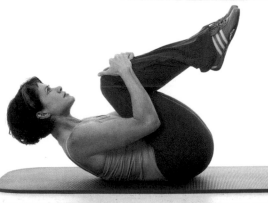

B Pull your abdominal muscles in and roll back onto your upper buttocks and lower back. Contract your abdominal muscles and pull yourself back to the start position. If the move is too difficult, loosen your arms, so your knees are pulled less tightly to your body.

Chapter 11

Detox! recipes
Food to make you feel great

Preparing food to detoxify your body should be a delightful adventure and these recipes will get you started. Optional or 'to taste' ingredients are not included in the nutritional analyses. If you prefer imperial measurements, use the conversion chart on page 185.

Apple pancakes

These ginger-spiced pancakes are terrific, and they're ready in just 20 minutes.

Makes 12 servings
115g wholemeal flour
115g plain white flour
40g fine cornmeal (polenta)
1 tbsp baking powder
1 tsp ground ginger
½ tsp bicarbonate of soda
450g virtually fat-free natural live yogurt
150ml skimmed milk
40g whole egg replacer
4 tbsp honey
2 tbsp rapeseed oil or other vegetable oil
1 apple, cored and grated
'light' oil cooking spray

1 In a blender or food processor, pulse the wholemeal and white flours, cornmeal, baking powder, ginger, bicarbonate of soda, yogurt, milk, egg replacer, honey and oil. (Alternatively, use 2 eggs instead of the egg replacer and omit the milk). Stir the apple into the batter.

2 Coat a large, non-stick frying pan with a 'light' olive oil or sunflower oil cooking spray and heat over a medium heat.

3 For each pancake, spoon 2 or 3 tablespoons of the batter into the frying pan. Cook until lightly browned and cooked through, about 2 minutes per side. Repeat with the remaining batter.

Detox! plus

Good for digestion • improving liver function • colon health

Apples contain pectin, a kind of water-soluble fibre that sweeps the intestines clean of toxins. **Wholemeal flour** and **cornmeal** are also rich in fibre.

Per serving 155kcals • 7g protein • 2g fat • 28g carbohydrate • 0.5mg cholesterol • 197mg sodium • 1g fibre

Berry morning crush

Low-fat cottage cheese provides a good supply of lean protein to help the liver carry out its detoxification duties; the fruit and nuts offer health-promoting antioxidants.

Makes 2 servings
225g low-fat natural live yogurt
2 tbsp honey
115g low-fat cottage cheese
115g blueberries and/or sliced strawberries
20g walnuts or almonds, crushed

1 Mix the yogurt, honey, cottage cheese, berries and nuts in a large bowl, then divide between two serving bowls.

Detox! plus

Good for • heart health • digestion

Cottage cheese is high in protein, which the body needs to do its detoxification work, and **walnuts** are rich in omega-3 fatty acids, good fats that combat heart disease. **Berries** are excellent sources of fibre and disease-fighting antioxidants.

Per serving • 229kcals • 15g protein • 9g fat • 24g carbohydrate • 4mg cholesterol • 247mg sodium • 1g fibre

Breakfast rice pudding

Eat dessert for breakfast – this family favourite is even healthier with tofu and brown rice.

Makes 4 servings
250g soft silken-style tofu
4 tbsp honey
2 tsp pure vanilla extract
½ tsp ground cinnamon
350g cooked brown rice
100g raisins
40g almonds

1 In a blender or food processor, blend the tofu with the honey, vanilla and cinnamon. Spoon into a bowl and add the rice, raisins and almonds. Mix well. Chill for several hours to blend the flavours.

Detox! plus

Good for • immune function • heart health • digestion

Tofu is a good source of zinc, necessary for good immune function, while **cinnamon** may help stop the growth of bacteria and fungi, including candida yeast. **Brown rice** is rich in fibre, which helps the body to eliminate toxins, as well as manganese, selenium and magnesium, enzymes that help in the detoxification process

Per serving • 367 kcals • 10g protein • 9g fat • 65g carbohydrate • 0mg cholesterol • 22mg sodium • 2g fibre

Apple pancakes

Fruited yogurt muesli

Natural yogurt comes alive with bursts of sweet and tangy flavour in this high-fibre treat.

Makes 4 servings
115g rolled oats
600ml water
1 tbsp virtually fat-free natural live yogurt
1 tbsp honey
2 tangerines, peeled and segmented
2 apples, chopped

1 In a large bowl, soak the oats in the water overnight, or let stand in the water for about 1 hour right before preparing. Stir in the yogurt, honey, tangerines and apples. Cover and chill any leftovers.

Detox! plus

Good for reducing candida yeast • improving liver function • colon health • digestion • lowering cholesterol

Live yogurt contains probiotics, good bacteria that take up residence in the intestine and protect the body from the bad bacteria and yeast overgrowth. **Tangerines** contain flavonoids, which help the liver to do its job of detoxifying the body. **Apples** and **rolled oats** contain fibre, which cleanses the digestive system, lowers cholesterol and protects heart health.

Per serving 166kcals • 4g protein • 3g fat • 33g carbohydrate • 1mg cholesterol • 13mg sodium • 3g fibre

Fruit melba breakfast sundae

Delicious fruit and nuts spooned over smooth and creamy yogurt.

Makes 2 servings
140g frozen raspberries, thawed
1 medium fruit of your choice (we suggest a ripe peach – unpeeled if organic, peeled if not – a banana or an orange)
150g virtually fat-free natural live yogurt
2 tbsp toasted flaked almonds

1 Place the raspberries in a food processor. Process until the berries form a smooth purée. Stone and slice the peach or other fruit. Divide the yogurt between two sundae glasses. Spoon the purée over the yogurt and top with the peach or other fruit. Sprinkle with the almonds.

Detox! plus

Good for heart health • digestion • bone health

Raspberries are rich in anthocyanins, plant chemicals with potent antioxidant powers, while **yogurt** is a good source of protein, B vitamins, and minerals, including calcium.

Per serving 139kcals • 8g protein • 6g fat • 14.5g carbohydrate • 0mg cholesterol • 64mg sodium • 3.5g fibre

Fruited yogurt muesli

Mandarin-kiwi fruit parfaits

Is it breakfast or is it dessert? It's good for you. It tastes scrumptious. Eat it anytime!

Makes 4 servings

450g virtually fat-free natural live yogurt
295g can mandarin oranges, drained
2 kiwi fruit, peeled, halved and sliced
4 ginger biscuits

1 In each of four parfait glasses, alternately layer the yogurt with the oranges and kiwi. Cover with cling film and chill until ready to serve. Serve with a ginger biscuit.

Fruit melba breakfast sundae

Detox! plus

Good for improving liver function • anti-ageing • colon health • reducing candida yeast

Kiwis and **mandarins** are both rich in vitamin C, an antioxidant that cleanses the body of harmful free radicals and so has an anti-ageing effect. **Mandarin oranges** also contain limonene, a nutrient that supports the liver's work of detoxifying the body. **Live yogurt** contains probiotics, good bacteria that prevent toxic bacteria and yeasts from growing in the intestines.

Per serving 133kcals • 7g protein • 2g fat • 24g carbohydrate • 1mg cholesterol • 117mg sodium • 1g fibre

Mexican red rice & beans

This spicy and flavour-packed dish is full of fibre.

Makes 2 servings
1 tsp olive oil
1 medium onion, chopped
½ garlic clove, crushed
200ml plus 1 tbsp water
100g brown basmati rice
230g can chopped tomatoes
1 small green pepper, chopped
¼ tsp chilli powder
¼ tsp dried oregano
¼ tsp ground cumin
1 or 2 drops hot pepper sauce
300g can low-salt kidney beans,
   drained and rinsed

1 In a large saucepan, combine the oil, onions, garlic and 1 tablespoon of the water. Cook over a medium heat, stirring frequently, for 6 to 7 minutes, or until the onions soften.

2 Add the rice, tomatoes, green pepper, chilli powder, oregano, cumin, hot pepper sauce and the remaining water. Stir, bring to the boil, then simmer for 25 minutes, or until the rice is tender and the liquid has been absorbed. Stir in the beans. Cook over a low heat for 2 minutes, or until heated through.

Detox! plus

Good for heart health • digestion • cancer protection

Tomatoes are a good source of vitamins A and C, and they contain the antioxidant lycopene, which helps to prevent cancer. **Kidney beans** contain fibre which aids digestion.

Per serving 339kcals • 13g protein • 4g fat • 67g carbohydrate • 0mg cholesterol • 68mg sodium • 10g fibre

Mexican red rice & beans

Fenugreek kichari

Kichari is a traditional Indian rice dish. Most variations are appropriate for use during semi-fasts. You can buy ghee in Indian speciality shops and many larger supermarkets. Or make your own by melting butter and carefully skimming off the foam. The clear oil that remains is the ghee, and it will keep in the fridge for several weeks.

Makes 4 servings
4 tbsp fenugreek seeds
400ml water
200g brown basmati rice
¼ tsp turmeric
½ tsp salt
3 tbsp ghee
I tbsp cumin seeds

1 Soak the seeds in the water overnight.

2 Put the rice in a pan with the seeds and water and bring to the boil. Add the turmeric and salt. Reduce the heat, cover and simmer over a low heat until all the water has been absorbed, about 25 minutes.

3 In a frying pan, heat the ghee and add the cumin seeds. Cover and remove from the heat. Let it stand for 15 to 30 seconds before adding to the cooked rice mixture.

Detox! plus

Good for fasting and cleansing

The **flavoured rice** in this dish is unlikely to provoke food sensitivities of any kind. It offers gentle nutritional support during a semi-fast.

Per serving 280kcals • 6g protein • 14g fat • 41g carbohydrate • 31.5mg cholesterol • 255mg sodium • Ig fibre

Barley with ginger & broccoli

This dish offers nutritional support to the liver without adding to its toxic burden.

Makes 2 servings
1.5 litres water
200g pearl barley (wholegrain)
2.5cm piece of fresh root ginger, sliced
I small head of broccoli, chopped into pieces
I tsp dried thyme
I½ tsp dried oregano
I½ tsp dried basil
Black pepper and ghee (optional)

1 Place the water, barley and ginger together in a medium saucepan, and bring to the boil. Lower the heat, cover the pan and let the mixture simmer for 35 minutes. Add the broccoli and continue to simmer until the barley is cooked, about 25 minutes more. Add the thyme, oregano, basil, black pepper, and ghee to taste if liked. Simmer a few minutes more, then serve.

Detox! plus

Good for fasting and cleansing • constipation • liver support

Broccoli contains sulphorophanes, biochemicals that the liver needs in order to carry out its work of detoxifying the body. Both **broccoli** and **barley** are high in fibre, which helps to reduce cholesterol while sweeping toxins from the body. This cleansing dish can be used during a semi-fast.

Per serving 326kcals • 14g protein • 3g fat • 65g carbohydrate • 0mg cholesterol • 10mg sodium • 17g fibre

Note Analysis does not include ghee, which can be added to taste.

Prawns with ginger, broccoli & corn

Exotic tasting yet easy-to-find flavourings make this stir-fry extra-special.

Makes 2 servings

140g broccoli florets
1½ tbsp reduced-salt soy sauce
1 tbsp rice vinegar
½ tbsp chopped fresh root ginger
¼ tsp chilli-garlic paste or purée
1¼ tsp toasted sesame oil
225g raw jumbo prawns, peeled and deveined
2 spring onions, thinly sliced
175g sweetcorn

1 Place the broccoli in a steamer, and gently steam over a low heat until crisp-tender, about 4 minutes. In a small bowl, whisk together the soy sauce, vinegar, ginger, chilli-garlic paste.

2 Just before serving, heat a wok or large non-stick frying pan over a high heat. Add the oil. When it ripples, add the prawns. Stir-fry for 2 to 3 minutes, or until the prawns are no longer translucent.

3 Add the broccoli, spring onions and sweetcorn, and then the soy mixture, and stir-fry until all the ingredients are coated with the sauce and heated through.

Detox! plus

Good for cancer protection • heart health • immune function

The main active components of **ginger**, gingerols, may inhibit the growth of cancer cells. Prawns are an excellent source of the mineral selenium, shown to protect cells from damage, support heart health and boost immunity.

Per serving 217kcals • 27g protein • 5g fat • 18g carbohydrate • 219mg cholesterol • 705mg sodium • 3g fibre

Prawns with ginger, broccoli & corn

Prawn tabbouleh

Adding prawns to this timeless Middle Eastern favourite turns it into a complete main dish.

Makes 4 servings
175g bulghur wheat
300ml boiling water
2 tbsp olive oil
450g prawns, cooked and peeled
1 cucumber, peeled and diced
1 medium red onion, finely chopped
30g fresh mint, snipped
30g fresh parsley, snipped
Juice of 1 lemon

1 Place the bulghur wheat in a large bowl and add the boiling water and oil. Cover and let stand for 30 minutes until the water has been absorbed.

2 Stir in the prawns, cucumber, onion, mint, parsley and lemon juice. Serve warm, or chill for at least an hour and serve cold.

Detox! plus

Good for digestion • colon and heart health • lowering cholesterol • improving liver function • anti-ageing

Parsley and **bulgur wheat** contain fibre to help to check excess cholesterol and aid digestion. **Parsley** is also rich in vitamin C, an anti-ageing, heart-protecting nutrient. **Onions** contain sulphur that the liver needs. It also needs the good quality protein in **prawns**.

Per serving 311kcals • 25g protein • 7g fat • 37g carbohydrate • 219mg cholesterol • 222mg sodium • 5g fibre

Chicken cassoulet

This elegant meal takes its name from a classic French recipe made with fatty duck meat and ham knuckles. Here it is made with chicken breasts and low-fat turkey boiling sausage.

Makes 4 servings

410g can cannellini beans in water,
    drained and rinsed

4 boneless, skinless chicken breasts

¼ tsp freshly ground black pepper

1 tbsp olive oil

175g smoked turkey or pork boiling sausage,
    thickly sliced

400ml low-salt chicken stock

1 medium onion, chopped

70g seasoned breadcrumbs

30g sun-dried tomatoes (not packed in oil),
    thinly sliced

2 tbsp chopped fresh basil, or 2 tsp dried

1 Preheat the oven to 180°C/ gas 4. Spread half of the beans in a 2 litre casserole.

2 Season the chicken with the pepper. In a large frying pan over a medium heat, brown the chicken in the oil for 5 minutes, turning once. Transfer the chicken to the casserole. Top with the sausage slices, remaining beans and stock.

3 In the same frying pan, cook the onions for 4 minutes, stirring to loosen any browned bits from the pan. Stir in the breadcrumbs, tomatoes and basil. Cook, stirring, for 2 minutes. Spread over the beans, patting to create a thick crust. Cover and bake for 10 minutes. Remove the cover and bake for a further 15 minutes or until the crust is browned. Serve.

Alternatively, the casserole can be frozen at this point. To serve, thaw in the fridge first, then reheat thoroughly in the oven.

Detox! plus

Good for improving liver function • anti-ageing • detoxifying the colon

Basil and **sun-dried tomatoes** are rich in body-protecting antioxidants. **Beans** are high in fibre, which helps to sweep waste from the body. **Chicken** and **turkey** are good sources of low-fat, high-quality protein to support the liver's detoxification efforts.

Per serving 399kcals • 48g protein • 13g fat • 25g carbohydrate • 105mg cholesterol • 716mg sodium • 4g fibre

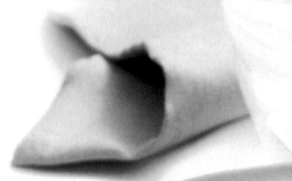

Chicken cassoulet

Chicken tamale pie

Tired of the same old chicken breast recipes? Try this spicy alternative. If you can't find egg substitute, use 1 egg instead.

Makes 4 servings
'light' oil cooking spray
350g boneless, skinless chicken breast, cubed
1 medium onion, chopped
1 tbsp chilli seasoning or 1 tsp chilli powder
400g can chopped tomatoes
175g sweetcorn
1 large green pepper, chopped
215g can kidney beans, drained and rinsed
1 tsp dried oregano
55g fine cornmeal (polenta)
70g plain white flour
1 tbsp sugar
1½ tsp baking powder
200ml skimmed milk
20g egg replacer or 1 medium egg

1 Preheat the oven to 200°C/gas 6. Coat a non-stick frying pan with a 'light' olive oil or sunflower oil cooking spray; heat for 1 minute. Add the chicken, onions and chilli powder. Cook, stirring often, until the chicken is browned and cooked through. Add the tomatoes, sweetcorn, pepper, beans and oregano, stirring to break up the tomatoes. Spoon into a 20cm square baking dish. At this point you can finish making the pie by covering the dish and baking for 10 minutes. Alternatively, cover it with foil and chill in the fridge until the next day.

2 Sift the cornmeal, flour, sugar and baking powder into a bowl. Blend the milk with the egg replacer (or lightly beat 1 egg with just 80ml of milk), pour into the bowl and mix with the dry ingredients to make a thick batter.

3 Spread the batter mixture evenly over the chicken and vegetables. Then return to the oven and bake for about 20 minutes, until a skewer inserted into the cornbread comes out clean.

Detox! plus

Good for detoxifying the colon • prostate health • improving liver function • anti-ageing

Peppers and **kidney beans** are high in fibre, which helps speed waste through the colon. **Green peppers** and **tomatoes** are high in vitamin C, an anti-ageing antioxidant. **Onions** contain sulphur and **chicken** has protein, both of which promote liver function.

Per serving 377kcals • 35g protein • 4g fat • 55g carbohydrate • 62mg cholesterol • 521mg sodium • 7g fibre

Red snapper Veracruz

Fish is always a heart-healthy choice – it is lower in fat than red meat and in any case its fats are the 'good' kind. With this lively, spicy dish, eating more fish is a pleasure.

Makes 4 servings
olive oil cooking spray
4 red snapper fillets (115g each)
1 tbsp lime juice
1 tsp dried oregano
2 tsp olive oil
1 onion, chopped
1 garlic clove, crushed
400g can tomatoes with pepper and chilli
12 pimiento-stuffed olives, coarsely chopped
2 tbsp chopped fresh parsley

1 Preheat the oven to 180°C/gas 4. Coat a square baking dish with olive oil cooking spray. Place the fillets in the baking dish. Sprinkle with the lime juice and oregano. Set aside.

2 Warm the oil in a medium frying pan over a medium heat. Add the onion and garlic. Cook, stirring occasionally, for 5 to 6 minutes until soft. Add the tomatoes, olives and parsley. Cook, stirring occasionally, for 5 minutes or until thickened. Spoon over the fillets. Cover tightly.

3 Bake for 18 to 20 minutes or until the fish flakes easily.

Detox! plus

Good for lowering cholesterol • arthritis • improving liver function • weight loss • prostate health

Fish oils have been shown to lower cholesterol. **Onions** contain sulphur, which helps to support the liver's detoxification efforts. **Tomatoes** contain lycopene, a phytochemical that helps to protect the prostate gland. This main course is also low in calories.

Per serving 158kcals • 24g protein • 4g fat • 6g carbohydrate • 43mg cholesterol • 332mg sodium • 2g fibre

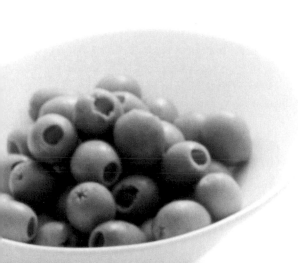

Red snapper Veracruz

Very vegetable omelette

The fresh vegetables in this quick-and-easy omelette provide flavour as well as plenty of fibre.

Makes 1 serving
olive oil cooking spray
2 eggs, well beaten
3 tbsp chopped red pepper
2 tbsp chopped green pepper
2 tbsp deseeded and chopped tomato
2 tbsp chopped courgette
2 tbsp chopped mushrooms (optional)
Salt and freshly ground black pepper

1 Coat a large frying pan with olive oil cooking spray and place it over a medium heat. When the pan is warm, add the eggs, allowing them to cover the bottom of the pan. Cook for 3 minutes, or until the bottom of the omelette begins to set.

2 When nearly cooked, top half of the omelette with the red and green peppers, tomato, courgette and mushrooms (if using) and season with salt and black pepper. Carefully fold the remaining half over the filling and cook for 2 minutes or until cooked right through.

Detox! plus

Good for improving liver function • heart health • cancer protection • digestion

Eggs are rich in choline, a substance that assists with the removal of fat in the liver. The **vegetables** provide fibre, which reduces the risk of heart disease and cancer and, in addition, the **peppers** are rich sources of the disease-fighting antioxidants vitamin C and beta-carotene.

Per serving 197kcals • 16g protein • 14g fat • 4g carbohydrate • 476mg cholesterol • 176mg sodium • 1g fibre

Aubergine bake with herb sauce

Bursting with the robust flavours of tomato, garlic, olive oil and herbs, this tofu-based bake tastes wonderfully decadent. Always wash vegetables well before cooking.

Makes 4 servings

280g firm silken-style tofu
500ml tomato passata
140g can tomato purée
1½ tbsp dried oregano
4 garlic cloves, crushed
freshly ground black pepper
3 medium courgettes
2 fresh medium tomatoes
1 medium aubergine
¼ tsp olive oil
1 medium onion, diced
6 slices wholegrain bread

1 Drain the tofu on a paper towel, then cut into 5mm slices. Preheat the oven to 180°C/gas 4. In a large mixing bowl, blend the passata, tomato purée, oregano and garlic and season to taste with black pepper. Set aside.

2 Cut the courgettes lengthways into 5mm slices. Cut the tomatoes and aubergine crossways into 5mm slices.

3 Rub the inside of a 3.5 litre casserole dish with the olive oil. Spread 4 tablespoons of the blended sauce in the bottom of the dish. Top with a layer of aubergine, then a layer of courgette. Scatter half the onion over the courgettes, then top evenly with the tofu and bread (the slices may overlap). Top the bread evenly with the tomato slices and half of the remaining sauce. Add the remaining onion, aubergine and courgette, then spread with the remaining sauce. Cover and bake for 45 to 50 minutes, or until the vegetables are tender when pierced with a fork. Remove the lid and allow the dish to stand at room temperature for 5 to 10 minutes before cutting. Serve hot.

Aubergine bake with herb sauce

Tuna tater

This good-for-you combination of lean protein (tuna and cheese) and healthy carbohydrates makes a delicious and satisfying meal.

Makes 1 serving
1 medium baking potato
140g frozen broccoli florets, thawed
80g tuna steak in spring water, drained
2 tbsp reduced-fat grated Cheddar-style cheese

1 Prick the potato with a fork, and microwave it on high for 8 minutes. In a medium microwave-safe bowl, microwave the broccoli on high for 4 minutes, then add the tuna. Cut the potato lengthways. Top with the tuna-broccoli mixture, then microwave on high for 1½ minutes. Sprinkle with the cheese.

Detox! plus

Good for heart health • cancer prevention

Potatoes are high in vitamin C, which combines with certain toxins in the body and destroys them. **Tuna** is rich in omega-3 fatty acids, which benefit the heart. **Broccoli** contains cancer-fighting isothiocyanates.

Per serving 305kcals • 36g protein • 5g fat • 30g carbohydrate • 52mg cholesterol • 428mg sodium • 6g fibre

Minestrone soup

There's no better way to eat your vegetables than by spooning up this rich and tasty soup.

Makes 4 servings
3 tbsp olive oil
1 leek, sliced
2 carrots, chopped
1 courgette, thinly sliced
115g green beans, cut into 2.5cm pieces
2 stalks celery, thinly sliced
1.5 litres vegetable stock
450g tomatoes, chopped
1 tbsp chopped fresh thyme
410g can cannellini beans in water
Salt and freshly ground black pepper

1 In a large saucepan, heat the olive oil over a medium heat. Add the sliced leek, carrots, courgette, green beans and celery. Cover, reduce the heat to low and cook for 15 minutes, shaking the pan occasionally. Stir in the stock, tomatoes and thyme. Bring to the boil. Cover and reduce the heat to low; simmer for 30 minutes. Stir in the cannellini beans, including the water. Simmer for an additional 10 minutes. Season with salt and pepper to taste before serving.

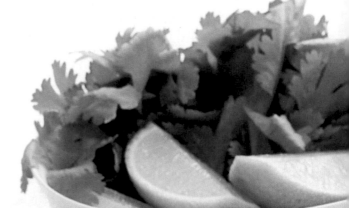

Detox! plus

Good for digestion • cancer prevention • heart health • cellular health

Cannellini beans are rich in heart-protective fibre. **Olive oil** is high in mono-unsaturated fat, which helps to lower cholesterol, and is rich in vitamins A, E and D. **Carrots** are rich in carotenoid antioxidants, which disarm free radicals that alter cells' DNA. **Celery** contains coumarins, compounds that help to prevent free radicals from damaging cells and so reduce the risk of cells becoming cancerous. A volatile oil in thyme, **thymol**, has anti-microbial effects, especially on the lungs.

Per serving 253kcals • 11g protein • 10g fat • 30g carbohydrate • 0mg cholesterol • 38mg sodium • 10g fibre

Tortilla soup with lime

Enjoy this satisfying soup with a green salad and you've done your body a double good turn.

Makes 4 servings

'light' oil cooking spray
4 corn tortillas (15cm in diameter),
   halved and cut into 5mm-wide strips
500ml chicken stock
300ml water
350g turkey breast slices, cut into
   1cm-thick strips
2 large onions, halved and thinly sliced
2 large red peppers, cut into thin strips
1 large jalapeño chilli, deseeded and finely
   chopped (wear plastic gloves when handling)
2 tsp ground cumin
¼ tsp dried oregano
85g frozen sweetcorn
75g cherry tomatoes, quartered
4 tbsp chopped fresh coriander
2 tbsp fresh lime juice
1 ripe avocado, diced

1 Preheat the oven to 200°C/gas 6. Coat one or two large baking sheets with 'light' olive oil or sunflower oil cooking spray.

2 Arrange the tortilla strips on the prepared baking sheets and bake for 2 minutes, or until crisped and lightly browned on the edges.

3 In a large saucepan, combine the stock, water, turkey, onions, peppers, chilli, cumin and oregano. Bring to the boil over high heat. Reduce the heat to medium-low, cover and simmer for 10 minutes.

4 Add the sweetcorn and simmer for 5 minutes. Stir in the tomatoes, coriander and lime juice. Ladle the soup into bowls and top each portion with avocado and tortilla crisps.

Detox! plus

Good for detoxifying from heavy metals • improving liver function • anti-ageing • prostate health

Coriander was shown in one small study to help to eliminate toxic heavy metal contamination from the body.

Per serving 441kcals • 30g protein • 13g fat • 54g carbohydrate • 50mg cholesterol • 213mg sodium • 7g fibre

Tortilla soup with lime

Emerald sesame greens

Kale, an under-estimated vegetable, has a deep, rich taste that goes well with ginger and sesame. Enjoy kale as a robust alternative to the milder taste of spinach.

Makes 4 servings

300g curly kale

½ tsp toasted sesame oil

½ tsp rapeseed or vegetable oil

I tsp crushed garlic

I tsp finely chopped fresh root ginger

I tbsp water

I tsp tamari or reduced-salt soy sauce

I tsp sesame seeds

¼ tsp cayenne pepper

1 Wash the kale but do not pat it dry. Chop it coarsely.

2 In a large non-stick frying pan or wok, warm the sesame and rapeseed oils over a medium-high heat. Add the garlic and ginger, and sauté until the garlic is lightly browned. Add the kale with the water that clings to it and sauté it, sprinkling with water as needed until it's tender, 5 to 7 minutes.

3 Transfer the kale to a bowl and toss with the tamari or soy sauce, sesame seeds and cayenne pepper.

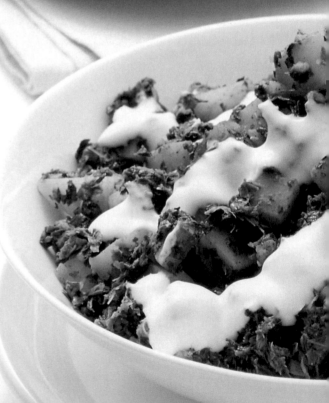

Indian-spiced potatoes & spinach

Indian-spiced potatoes & spinach

Potatoes as a side dish are all too often 'ho-hum'. In this dish, they positively sing with flavour. And it's always a good idea to incorporate turmeric into your diet. Not only a tasty spice, it's also a powerful detoxifying herb.

Makes 4 servings

2 medium Desirée potatoes, peeled, scrubbed and cut into 1cm chunks
2 tbsp rapeseed oil
3 garlic cloves, crushed
1 medium onion, chopped
1¾ tsp ground cumin
¾ tsp ground coriander
½ tsp ground turmeric
½ tsp ground cinnamon
¼ tsp ground ginger
¼ tsp salt
¼ tsp freshly ground black pepper
450g frozen cut-leaf spinach
2–4 tbsp water
150g virtually fat-free natural live yogurt

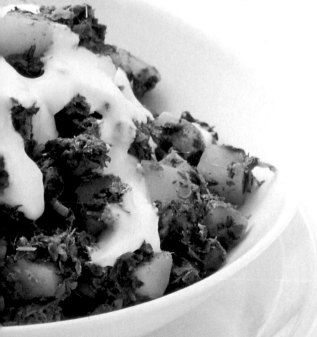

1 Place a steamer basket in a large saucepan with 125ml of water. Place the potatoes in the steamer. Bring to the boil over a high heat. Reduce the heat to medium, cover and cook for 20 minutes, or until the potatoes are very tender.

2 Place the potatoes in a bowl and keep warm. Drain and dry the saucepan. Heat the oil in the same saucepan over a medium heat. Add the garlic and onion and cook, stirring frequently, for 5 minutes or until soft. Add the cumin, coriander, turmeric, cinnamon, ginger, salt and pepper and cook, stirring, for 30 seconds to cook the spices.

3 Add the potatoes and cook, stirring frequently, for 5 minutes or until coated and flavoured with the spice mixture.

4 Add the spinach and 2 tablespoons of water. Cover and cook, tossing gently. Add additional water, 1 tablespoon at a time, if needed, for 5 minutes or until heated through. Place in a serving bowl. Drizzle the yogurt on top, but don't stir it in. Serve hot.

Detox! plus

Good for improving liver function • intestinal health • eliminating candida yeast

Turmeric helps the liver to balance the different aspects of its efforts, shortening the transit time for the worst chemical by-products of detoxification. **Live yogurt** contains probiotics, the good kind of bacteria that promote better digestion, prevent candida yeast overgrowth and keep the intestines healthy.

Per serving 180kcals • 8g protein • 7g fat • 23.5g carbohydrate • 0mg cholesterol • 315mg sodium • 4g fibre

Barley salad with smoked cheese

Smoky Gouda cheese, garlic and olive oil, as well as a variety of vegetables, turn barley into a surprisingly satisfying salad.

Makes 2 servings

200g pearl barley

2 tbsp balsamic vinegar

2 tbsp virtually fat-free natural live yogurt

½ tbsp olive oil

1 garlic clove, crushed

pinch of salt (optional)

freshly ground black pepper

1 small red onion, chopped

4 tbsp chopped fresh parsley

2 spring onions, chopped

150g cherry tomatoes, halved

2 carrots, grated

80g smoked Gouda cheese, cubed

Detox! plus

Good for heart health • improving liver function • digestion

Barley is a good source of soluble fibre, which can help to lower levels of total cholesterol. It also contains vitamin E which protects against toxic free radicals in the liver, and beta glucans, a specific type of soluble fibre that helps to prevent dietary fats and cholesterol from being absorbed by the intestines.

Per serving 608kcals • 22g protein • 17g fat • 96g carbohydrate • 34mg cholesterol • 426mg sodium • 3g fibre

---

1 Place the barley in a large saucepan. Add cold water to cover. Bring to the boil. Cook for 10 minutes, or until the barley is soft but not mushy. Drain, rinse to remove excess starch, drain again and set aside to cool.

2 In a medium salad bowl, whisk together the vinegar, yogurt, oil, garlic, salt (if using) and pepper to taste. Stir in the red onion, parsley and spring onions. Add the tomatoes, carrots, Gouda and barley. Toss to mix well.

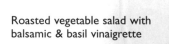

Roasted vegetable salad with balsamic & basil vinaigrette

Roasted vegetable salad with balsamic & basil vinaigrette

Eating your vegetables has never been this easy. You'll love this hearty salad of aubergine, tomato, courgette, pepper and onion, all tossed with a piquant vinaigrette dressing.

Makes 2 servings

1 tbsp balsamic vinegar
1 garlic clove, crushed
¾ tsp dried basil
1½ tbsp plus 2 tsp olive oil
1 red onion, quartered and
   separated into 'petals'
1 medium courgette, cubed
½ small aubergine, cubed
1 red pepper, thinly sliced
1 medium tomato, cut
   into wedges
¼ tsp fennel seeds, crushed
pinch of freshly ground black pepper

1 In a small bowl, whisk together the vinegar, garlic, ¼ teaspoon of the basil and 1½ tablespoons of the oil. Set aside. Preheat the oven to 230°C/gas 8. Coat a 33 x 23cm baking dish with 1 teaspoon of the remaining oil.

2 In a medium bowl, toss the onion, courgette, aubergine, red pepper, tomato, fennel seeds, black pepper, the remaining ½ teaspoon of basil and the remaining teaspoon of oil. Place in the baking dish. Roast, stirring occasionally, for 20 to 30 minutes, or until the vegetables are tender. Transfer to a large bowl. Serve warm or chilled. Toss with the basil vinaigrette just before serving.

Detox! plus

Good for heart health • cancer prevention

The **vegetables** are high in fibre and various antioxidants, which help to neutralise and destroy free radicals that can lead to heart disease, cancer and other diseases. **Basil** contains monoterpenoids, compounds with antibacterial properties.

Per serving 181kcals • 3.5g protein • 12g fat • 15g carbohydrate • 0mg cholesterol • 11mg sodium • 4g fibre

Fresh fruit salad with almonds

A simple but satisfying way to get a daily dose of fibre. The lime and mint add a burst of flavour.

Makes 2 servings

350g assorted chopped or sliced fresh fruit (such as apples, oranges, bananas, grapes and blueberries)
juice of ½ lime
½ tsp finely chopped fresh mint
1 tbsp crushed almonds

1 Put the fruit in a large bowl. Add the lime juice and mint; toss gently to coat. Sprinkle with the crushed almonds.

Detox! plus

Good for digestive health • heart health • cancer protection

Fruit is bursting with soluble fibre, which helps the body to eliminate toxins and promotes weight loss, thereby helping to protect against heart disease. **Almonds** are rich in vitamin E, which some studies suggest may protect against cervical and prostate cancers.

Per serving 125kcals • 2g protein • 3g fat • 23.5g carbohydrate • 0mg cholesterol • 6mg sodium • 3g fibre

Mandarin cabbage slaw

What could be easier than this delicious, healthy salad? Once you've shredded the cabbage, you just fold it all together.

Makes 4 servings

200g white cabbage, shredded
400g can hearts of palm, drained and cut into strips
295g can mandarin oranges, drained
5 tbsp low-fat vinaigrette dressing

1 In a large bowl, combine the cabbage, hearts of palm and mandarins. Toss with the dressing.

Detox! plus

Good for weight loss • colon health • improving liver function • lowering cholesterol • cancer prevention

Cabbage is one of the cruciferous vegetables, all of which contain powerful anti-cancer compounds. **Cabbage** is also high in fibre, which helps to sweep wastes from the body and lowers cholesterol.

Per serving 58.5kcals • 3g protein • 1g fat • 12g carbohydrate • 0mg cholesterol • 507mg sodium • 2.5g fibre

Mediterranean coleslaw

Mediterranean coleslaw

This coleslaw is a refreshing change from commercial coleslaw, which is typically made with mayonnaise and sugar. Enjoy this side dish at your next outdoor barbecue or the next time you bring home a ready-cooked roast chicken.

Makes 4 servings
2 medium tomatoes
200g white cabbage, shredded
1 red pepper, finely sliced
4 tbsp olive oil
juice from ½ lemon
½ tsp salt (or to taste)

1 Quarter and slice the tomatoes very thinly. They will release a lot of juice as you slice them. Combine that juice, the tomato slices, the cabbage and the sliced pepper in a bowl. Drizzle on the olive oil and toss. Add the lemon juice and salt and toss again.

2 You can eat this right away, but it's even better after a couple of hours or even the next day. If you wait until the next day, you may find that you need to add a little more lemon juice to moisten. You can use green pepper instead of red, if that's what you have on hand, but the red pepper is prettier in this dish.

Detox! plus

Good for detoxifying the colon • improving liver function • heart health • constipation

Tomatoes and **red peppers** are high-antioxidant foods. This slaw is also a high-fibre food that encourages the swift movement of food through the digestive system. **Cabbage** contains sulphoraphane, a biochemical that the liver needs in order to carry out its detoxification efforts. All the **vegetables** contain vitamin C, a heart-protective antioxidant. And the **olive oil** is mono-unsaturated, a type of oil that helps to keep your cholesterol levels under control.

Per serving 136kcals • 2g protein • 11g fat • 7g carbohydrate • 0mg cholesterol • 10mg sodium • 3g fibre

Moroccan carrot salad with toasted cumin

Carrots are a traditional choice for detoxifying the body. Eating more carrots is always a good idea, and when they taste this good, who can resist?

Makes 4 servings

¾ tsp ground cumin
¼ tsp ground coriander
142ml carton low fat soured cream
   (or half-fat crème fraîche)
4 tsp lemon juice
1½ tsp extra-virgin olive oil
1½ tsp flaxseed oil
¼ tsp freshly grated orange peel
¼ tsp salt
7 medium carrots, grated
125g currants
½ small red onion, thinly sliced

1 In a small frying pan over a medium heat, cook the cumin and coriander, stirring often, for 2 minutes or until fragrant and slightly darker in colour.

2 Place in a medium bowl and let cool. Stir in the soured cream, lemon juice, olive oil, flaxseed oil, orange zest and salt.

3 Add the carrots, currants and onion and toss to coat well. Let stand for 15 minutes to allow the flavours to blend.

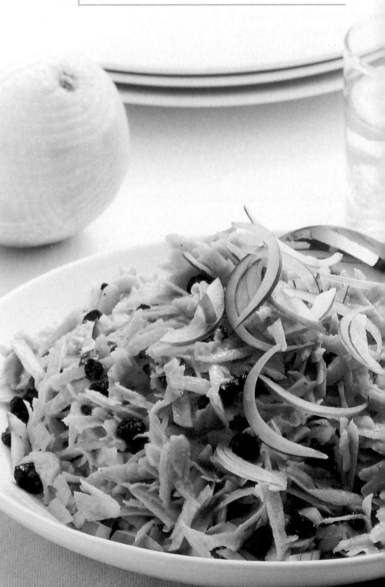

Garlic-herb dip

You'll love dipping crudités into this tasty dip, enlivened with fresh dill and parsley.

Makes 6 servings (2 tablespoons each)
142ml carton soured cream
4 tbsp mayonnaise
2 large garlic cloves, crushed
1 tbsp chopped fresh parsley
1 tbsp Worcestershire sauce
½ tbsp finely chopped onion
½ tbsp chopped fresh dill
½ tsp salt

1 In a small bowl, thoroughly combine the soured cream, mayonnaise, garlic, parsley, Worcestershire sauce, onion, dill and salt.

Detox! plus

Good for eye health • cancer prevention

Garlic contains quercetin, an antioxidant shown to protect colon cells from certain cancer-causing substances. **Parsley** contains terpenoids, compounds that have an anti-cancer effect. **Dill** is a good source of beta-carotene and a fair source of lutein and zeaxanthin, all of which help to protect eyesight.

Per serving 124kcals • 1g protein • 12.5g fat • 2g carbohydrate • 22.5mg cholesterol • 249mg sodium • 1g fibre

Turkish white-bean dip

Serve this creamy dip with tortilla chips, pitta bread, raw vegetables or oatcakes.

Makes 10 servings (2 tablespoons each)
410g can white beans, such as cannellini, in water, drained and rinsed
2 tsp extra-virgin olive oil
2 tsp lime juice
1 tsp ground cumin
1 tsp crushed garlic
50g rocket or watercress, chopped
salt and freshly ground black pepper

1 In a food processor or blender, combine the beans, oil, lime juice, cumin and garlic. Process until smooth.

2 Transfer to a small bowl. Stir in the rocket or watercress and season to taste.

Detox! plus

Good for detoxifying the colon • lowering cholesterol • heart health • weight loss

Beans are high in fibre, which speeds waste removal from the colon and helps to lower cholesterol. **Fibre** also provides a feeling of fullness that satisfies the appetite.

Per serving 32kcals • 2g protein • 1g fat • 4g carbohydrate • 0mg cholesterol • 2mg sodium • 1g fibre

Morrocan carrot salad with toasted cumin

Salted edamame

Edamame are soyabeans harvested while they're still green, just before they've had a chance to harden. They are hailed as a super-food, and are enjoyed as a snack in Asia, particularly in Japan. You can buy them frozen from Asian stores, or on the internet.

Makes 8 servings
450g fresh or frozen unshelled edamame
½ tsp coarse salt

1 Bring a large pan of water to a boil over a high heat. Add the edamame and cook until bright green and tender, about 10 minutes for fresh or 5 minutes for frozen. Remove the edamame from the boiling water with a slotted spoon and place in a bowl of iced water. Drain well.

2 Place the edamame in a serving bowl and toss with the salt. To eat, pop open the shells and slip the edamame into your mouth. Serve with a bowl for empty shells.

Detox! plus

Good for cancer prevention • relieving premenstrual and menopausal symptoms • improving liver function • weight loss

Edamame is rich in isoflavones, compounds that mimic oestrogen. Because they take the place of oestrogen in the body, isoflavones are believed to help to prevent conditions associated with excess oestrogen, among them breast cancer and PMS and menopausal discomforts caused by low oestrogen. **Edamame** also contains a complete protein, which means that it is a good choice for vegetarians looking to support the liver's detoxification efforts.

Per serving 80 kcals • 6g protein • 2.5g fat • 4g carbohydrate • 0mg cholesterol • 140mg sodium • 3g fibre

Tahini dressing

Given bite with garlic, tahini and cayenne pepper, this intensely flavoured dressing will make otherwise plain vegetables dramatic.

Makes 2 servings
150g virtually fat-free natural live yogurt
1 garlic clove, crushed
3 tbsp tahini (sesame seed paste)
1 tbsp lemon juice
1 tsp ground cumin
½ tsp salt
¼ tsp ground cayenne pepper

1 Whisk the yogurt, garlic, tahini, lemon juice, cumin, salt and pepper in a bowl until smooth.

Detox! plus

Good for digestion

Cayenne pepper stimulates circulation, aids digestion and promotes sweating, all of which aid the body's detoxification's efforts. **Cumin** may stimulate the secretion of pancreatic enzymes necessary for proper digestion and the assimilation of nutrients. **Tahini** is a good source of copper and thiamin, a B vitamin that helps to convert food into energy.

Per serving 179kcals • 8g protein • 13g fat • 7g carbohydrate • 1mg cholesterol • 549mg sodium • 2g fibre

Tomato & dill dressing

Tahini is a paste made of ground sesame seeds; tamari is a rich, dark soy sauce. Together, they lend a hint of smoky flavour to the tomatoes and dill in this delicious dressing.

Makes 8 servings (2 tablespoons each)

175ml tahini

3 tbsp tamari

7 garlic cloves

4 tomatoes

125ml water

½ tbsp chopped fresh dill

1 Blend the tahini, tamari, garlic, tomatoes, water and dill in a food processor until creamy.

Detox! plus

Good for immune function • cancer prevention

Garlic contains essential oils and other components that have potent antibiotic, antifungal and antiviral properties. **Dill** contains volatile oils that may help to neutralise such carcinogens as the benzopyrenes in cigarette smoke.

Per serving 146kcals • 5g protein • 13g fat • 2.5g carbohydrate • 0mg cholesterol • 330mg sodium • 2g fibre

Sunflower seed dressing

Fresh herbs add zing – and health benefits – to this 'sunny' dressing.

Makes 12 servings (4 tablespoons each)

200g sunflower seeds

450ml water

125ml lemon juice

2 tbsp tamari

2 tbsp honey

1 tsp salt

½ green pepper, deseeded

20g fresh basil, chopped

20g fresh coriander, chopped

1 Process the sunflower seeds, water, lemon juice, tamari, honey, salt, pepper, basil and coriander in a food processor until creamy.

Detox! plus

Good for heart health • bone health

The **sunflower seeds** contain linoleic acid, which can help to reduce cholesterol deposits on the walls of the arteries.

Per serving 112kcals • 4g protein • 8g fat • 7g carbohydrate • 0mg cholesterol • 308mg sodium • 1g fibre

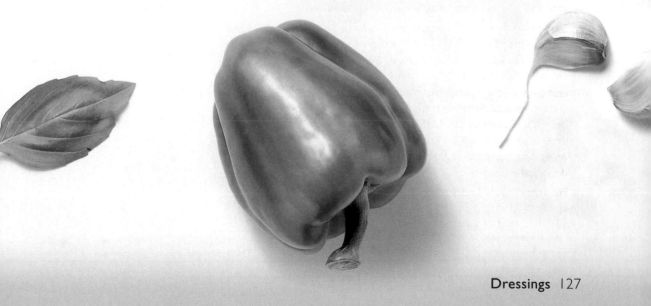

Rice protein shake

Protein plays a vital role in detoxification, and this rich shake is full of it, as well as healthy fats and antioxidants.

Makes 1 serving
225ml rice milk
1 scoop (25g) skimmed milk powder
1 tbsp flax oil
115g berries or ½ sweet potato
1 tbsp wheatgerm or honey (optional)

1 Whizz the rice milk, milk powder, oil and berries or sweet potato in a blender until smooth. Add the wheatgerm or honey (if using).

Detox! plus

Good for improving liver function

Flax oil is rich in essential fatty acids, which support liver detoxification. **Wheat germ** aids digestion by adding fibre. **Berries** are rich in vitamin C. Sweet potato contains chemicals which help to clear the body of toxic heavy metals.

Per serving 297kcals • 18g protein • 12g fat • 32g carbohydrate • 11mg cholesterol • 240mg sodium • 2g fibre

Note Analysis does not include optional wheatgerm or honey.

Carrot-apple snazz

This juice is sweet, tart and slightly astringent at the same time. Use this satisfying drink as a meal replacement while fasting, or enjoy it as a refresher at any time.

Makes 1 serving
4 carrots, peeled
1 apple, peeled, cored and cut into chunks
handful of parsley
2 stalks celery

1 Alternately, feed the carrots and apple chunks into the juicer. Then add the parsley and celery and blend together.

Detox! plus

Good for fasting and cleansing • improving liver function • heart health • antiageing

The **fruit and vegetable juices** contain nutrients that can support liver function while you're fasting and cleansing. They are also rich in antioxidants, which help to protect the heart and have an anti-ageing effect.

Per serving 165kcals • 3g protein • 1g fat • 38g carbohydrate • 0mg cholesterol • 137mg sodium • 10.5g fibre

Fruit smoothie

Filled with fibre and plant protein, this creamy treat is as healthy as it is delicious.

Makes 1 serving

225ml skimmed or soya milk
125 to 225ml water
115g berries, mashed banana or other fruit
1 scoop (25g) skimmed milk powder
1 tbsp wheatgerm or honey (optional)

1 Whizz the milk, water, fruit and milk powder in a blender until smooth. Add the wheatgerm or honey (if using).

Detox! plus

Good for breast health • improving liver function • digestion • heart health

Soya milk is high in phytoestrogens (a natural form of oestrogen found in plants), which may help to protect against breast cancer. The fibre, vitamins, minerals and plant compounds in fruit support liver detoxification.

Per serving 273kcals • 18g protein • 1g fat • 51g carbohydrate • 11mg cholesterol • 238mg sodium • 1g fibre

Note Analysis does not include optional wheatgerm or honey.

Peach, apple & pear surprise

The surprise is how easy it is to get the benefits of four pieces of fruit in just one glass – and also how good it tastes.

Makes 1 serving

2 peaches, stones removed
1 apple, cored and sliced
1 pear, cored and sliced

1 Process the peaches, apple and pear in a juicer and serve.

Detox! plus

Good for improving liver function • fasting and cleansing • weight loss • lowering cholesterol • heart health • anti-ageing

Peaches contain carotenes and flavonoids, which support the liver's detoxifying efforts. **Apples** and **pears** both contain pectin, a type of water-soluble fibre, much of which is still present when the fruit is juiced. **Fibre** helps to sweep wastes from the colon and lower cholesterol.

Per serving 184kcals • 3g protein • 0.5g fat • 45g carbohydrate • 0mg cholesterol • 10mg sodium • 9g fibre

Orange, mango and kiwi juice

Sparkling mineral water adds zest to this invigorating fruit juice.

Makes 1 serving
1 orange, peeled and segmented
½ mango, peeled, stoned and sliced
1 kiwi fruit, peeled and sliced
Sparkling mineral water

1 Process the orange, mango and kiwi in a juicer. Pour the juice into a large glass. Top up with mineral water and serve.

Detox! plus

Good for fasting and cleansing • improving liver function • anti-ageing • colds

Oranges contain limonene, a phytochemical that the liver needs in order to carry out its detoxification of the body. **Orange**, **mango** and **kiwi** are all high in vitamin C, an anti-ageing nutrient and a powerful antioxidant.

Per serving 131kcals • 3g protein • 1g fat • 31g carbohydrate • 0mg cholesterol • 12mg sodium • 6g fibre

Vegetable juice

Start your day with this low-calorie, delicious and nutritious juice.

Makes 1 serving
225ml water
1 beetroot, peeled and finely chopped
2 carrots, peeled and finely chopped
3 leaves fresh spinach, washed and finely chopped, about 30g in total
2 tomatoes, skinned if liked and finely chopped
fresh lime juice (add a few drops first and then check to see if you need more)
salt and freshly ground black pepper, to taste

1 Process the water, beetroot, carrots, spinach, tomatoes and lime juice in a blender until smooth. Season to taste and serve immediately.

Detox! plus

Good for fasting and cleansing • improving liver function • prostate health • weight loss • heart health

Tomatoes supply vitamin C, carotenes, potassium and lycopene, which protects the prostate. **Carrots** have carotenes, as well. The liver needs a variety of carotenes in order to detoxify the body.

Per serving 110kcals • 4g protein • 1g fat • 22g carbohydrate • 0mg cholesterol • 130mg sodium • 7g fibre

Chapter 12
Home treatments
Setting up your home spa

At one time spas were only for the idle rich. Not so anymore. Day spas can be found just about anywhere, making access to a spa experience easier than ever. You can even do some of the treatments at home.

Thanks to the internet and health-minded consumers, the companies that furnish luxurious commercial spas with their 'magic formulas' have made it possible to have a spa experience in the privacy of your own home.

In addition to online sources, spa-type treatment essentials can be found anywhere from cosmetics counters and natural product boutiques to ordinary supermarket shelves and health-food shops. Some of the 'magic' found in certain spa formulas can even be found on your kitchen shelves. The result is a wealth of options that leave you with only one big question: where to begin?

The ultimate benefits of a spa experience are the nature-based therapies that detoxify and purify the body. Modern everyday living makes the body a magnet for toxins. Spas use special ingredients from nature that are rich in minerals that have the ability to pull impurities out of the body.

Creating ambience

The common denominator in any spa experience is the expulsion of stress, which is in itself toxic. And, to this end, spas go to great lengths to create a stress-free atmosphere.

In the home, the focal point of the personal spa is the bathroom. Most bathrooms are not big enough to accommodate a chair, let alone a recliner, and bathroom fittings are not exactly like furniture when it comes to rearranging. Yet there is much you can do to create enough ambience for a convincing 'spa' feel.

Depending on the size of your bathroom, bring a plant or two into the room or, if you prefer, fresh flowers. Dim the light or buy floating, perfumed candles. Check the list of mood-altering aromatics and essences in 'Add oils to boost the bath' on page 133.

Invest in a luxurious robe that wraps around you generously, as well as extra-soft, extra-large bath towels. Add to the atmosphere with soothing music. Indulge in some luxury accessories such as a loofah, a long-handled bristle brush for your back, a sea sponge, gel eye masks, bath oils, lotions and fine soaps. Have plenty of iced spring or mineral water on hand and set a dish of detoxifying freshly sliced lemons next to it.

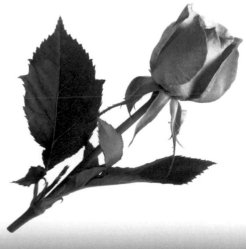

The purifying treatments in this chapter use the following household items. Keep them in your refrigerator or cupboard.

- Aloe vera gel
- Baking soda
- Cider vinegar
- Epsom salts
- Fresh flowers
- Herbal teas
- Lemons
- Mineral water
- Mist bottle
- Muslin
- Natural bristle brush
- Olive oil
- Powdered milk
- Rolled oats
- Sea salt
- Spring water
- Teabags or tea infusor

Soak some weed

When it comes to whole-body detoxifiers, seaweed is believed to be the most potent. Combined with the heat of bathwater, the minerals in seaweed penetrate the skin through the pores and draw out the impurities. A special kind of seaweed called spirulina, or blue-green algae, has the ability to purify to the deepest levels of the body.

Seaweed comes in thousands of species and in a variety of colours and textures, and contains large amounts of minerals such as calcium, phosphorous, magnesium, iron, iodine and sodium, though the amounts can vary from type to type. They also contain acids that bind with toxins and expel them from the body. Therapeutic seaweed comes in both powder and dried form. For a more realistic feel, you can purchase a gel that you can rub directly on your skin. Just be sure to follow the product directions. Before you take your first plunge, remember these points.

Contain yourself You don't want the remnants of your seaweed bath to go down the drain, so you'll need to steep dried seaweed in an infusion ball or muslin bag, in hot water for 20 to 30 minutes. As you are running the bath, toss the infusion ball or bag into the tub along with the steeped hot water.

Make it hot Because toxins exit the body through perspiration, you should make the bath as hot as you safely can stand it. A slight film will form on your skin as the seaweed coats it. Once your skin absorbs the seaweed, the film will disappear. This tells you that it is time to get out of the bath.

Take a plunge To get the total detoxifying effect, dip down deep into the water so that your shoulders are covered.

Take care If the bath makes you dizzy or light-headed, get out at once. Also, if you have high blood pressure, heart disease or are being treated for any chronic ailment, check with your doctor before taking a seaweed bath.

Playing with mud & clay

Sea muds and clays are also common spa detoxifying agents. Mud masks help to pull the impurities out from the skin. Clay treatments are much more specialized.

Clays are commonly used for facial masks, body wraps and baths, and as carriers for aromatherapy formulas. It works by generating heat that draws toxins out of the body and absorbing oils, dirt and bacteria from the skin's surface. It also pulls moisture and oil from the skin, so you don't want to use it if you have dry or dehydrated skin.

Clays and muds are simple to use. Select a product that appeals to you and follow the

ADD OILS TO BOOST THE BATH

Essential oils are natural substances extracted from flowers, herbs, fruits, trees and grasses through a special distilling process. Many of these oils have been found to contain healing properties. Some are also known to affect the nervous system, to calm or stimulate. Remember that essential oils are potent and that a drop or two is sufficient. They should never be used directly on the skin; try to keep them away from your mouth, nose, eyes and vagina, and never take them internally.

ESSENCES THAT SOOTHE

Basil Helps to ease muscle aches and pains. It is also used in skin toners.

Bergamot Possesses antitoxin agents. Effective against acne and blemishes. *Caution:* Do not expose skin to the sun after using it.

Cedarwood Possesses antitoxin agents. Good for oily skin.

Chamomile Helps skin conditions such as dermatitis, psoriasis, acne and herpes.

Clary sage Good for treating ageing skin and varicose veins.

Cypress Helps to alleviate bruising, muscle cramps and broken capillaries. Believed to help to control cellulite.

Geranium Helps to ease breast tenderness and swelling.

Hyssop Helps to ease dermatitis, eczema and acne, and to reduce water retention.

Jasmine A softener for dry, sensitive skin. Also believed to have aphrodisiac qualities.

Lavender Helps to soothe inflamed skin.

Mandarin Good for scars and stretch marks. A great skin toner. *Caution:* Do not expose skin to the sun after using it.

Marjoram Has extra-strength calming qualities.

Neroli Good for scars, stretch marks, sensitive and ageing skin.

Patchouli Helps to soothe skin irritations. Good for ageing skin and varicose veins.

Peppermint Soothes muscle aches and pains. Helps to constrict capillaries.

Rose Good for ageing skin. Believed to have aphrodisiac qualities.

Sandalwood Good for dry and ageing skin. Believed to have aphrodisiac qualities.

ESSENCES THAT ENERGIZE

Eucalyptus Possesses antitoxin qualities. Helps to heal blisters and other skin irritations.

Ginger Helps to fight congestion; improves circulation. *Caution:* Do not use on sensitive skin.

Grapefruit Helps to fight muscle fatigue and jet lag. Noted for its cleansing effect on the circulatory and lymphatic systems. Also good for oily skin. *Caution:* Do not expose skin to the sun after using it.

Juniper Known as a detoxifying agent. Also good for oily skin and blocked pores.

Lemon Helps to lighten skin pigmentation. *Caution:* Do not expose skin to the sun after using it.

Lemongrass Eases muscle soreness, bruising, and athlete's foot. Good for ageing skin.

Pine Helps to fight eczema and psoriasis. *Caution:* Do not use on sensitive skin.

Rosemary Eases sore muscles. Good for oily skin.

directions on the package. Apply it generously to your face in small, circular motions. Leave it on for 10 to 15 minutes. Remove the mud with warm water and a washcloth. To enhance the experience, you can also do the following:

Add some essence Instead of using mineral water, use a floral water made from any of the essences recommended in 'Add oils to boost the bath' on the previous page. Or add 2 or 3 drops of an aromatherapy oil.

Be still Lie back, close your eyes, put on some soft music and relax. You want your facial muscles to relax, so let the mask do its magic by being as still as possible.

Play misty You do not want the mask to dry out before your 15 minutes are up. If you feel it beginning to crack, spray your face with a water mist, or a mist fragranced with a few drops of aromatherapy oil. Keep your mister beside you so you can grab it without moving too much.

Steam first Steaming before you apply a mask will help to increase the effectiveness of the mask by opening the pores so dirt and impurities can escape. To steam properly and safely, do the following:

1 **Heat** a pot of water on the stove until the water is simmering but not boiling.

2 **Pour** the water into a ceramic bowl that is sitting on a nonslip surface. Fill the bowl to no more than 2.5cm (1in) from the top.

3 **Drape** a towel over your head to make a tent, close your eyes, and place your face 20cm to 25cm (8in to 10in) above the water. If the water gets too hot, lift the end of the towel to release some heat. Carefully steam for 5 minutes.

Refresh By the end of the mask, your pores will be tightened and your face will feel soft. Gently spray your face with the purified mist you have handy and let it dry.

Go for it all Do a detoxifying mask and bath at the same time.

A cucumber makes it complete About the only body parts not accounted for, at this point, are the eyes. Put a slice of cucumber or a wet teabag on each eyelid to help to pull out built-up fluid and reduce swelling. Some women prefer to wear a gel mask, which has the same effect.

Salts of the sea & other purifiers

Celtic Sea and Dead Sea salts are used in spas because they have a high mineral content and are slightly moist. Household Epsom salts have similar qualities. Therapeutic salts should not be confused with common table salt that offers no healing qualities.

Salts have detoxifying qualities because they encourage perspiration. Like clays and muds, they leave your skin feeling silky.

Baking soda, also known as bicarbonate of soda, is highly alkaline and has been found to help to leach from your system toxins caused by pollution, cigarettes and alcohol. Baking soda is commonly combined with sea salts to make formulas for detox baths. Making a detoxifying bath using sea salts is easy. Just combine the following:

You will need 1 cup of Dead Sea, Celtic Sea or any marine sea salts (you can also combine different salts), 1 cup Epsom salts and 2 cups baking soda.

Make a large batch of the salt solution and keep it in a jar with a tight lid. At bath time, add about ¼ cup of the salts to the bath as you are running the water in.

To enhance the experience, make the bath as hot as possible. Add a few drops of essential oils to the bath. To enhance the detoxifying effect, add a tablespoon of powdered seaweed to the bath while you're running the water. Mixing hydrogen peroxide into the bath creates a concentration of oxygen that stimulates the circulatory and lymphatic systems. The water needs to be hot in order to create perspiration.

Fancy footwork

Sea salts are also great for soothing tired and aching feet and for softening calluses. Put sea salts in a large bowl of tepid water with a few drops of rosemary, peppermint and lavender essential oils to help stimulate circulation. To pamper your feet further:

Add some comfort Take your footbath while sitting in the comfort of your favourite chair.

Roll around Put 8 to 10 equal-size marbles in the footbath and roll your feet over them while you're soaking. The marbles will give you a mini-massage.

Do a scrub instead Rather than a bath, make a scrub by mixing the salts and essential oils with enough olive oil to make a paste and vigorously rub it into your feet. Put your feet up, lean back and relax for 15 minutes. Rinse your feet clean.

Have heat waiting Before either the bath or the scrub, put a big, fluffy towel in the clothes dryer and time it to come out as your treatment ends. Wrap your feet up in the warmth and relax for another 5 minutes or so.

Whole-body treatments

The skin is not only the largest human organ, it is the only organ exposed directly to the pollution, dirt and chemicals that we encounter on a daily basis. In addition to serving as an outlet for body toxins, it also has its own waste product to deal with – dead skin.

Sloughing away dead skin, also known as exfoliating, should be part of your daily detoxifying ritual. A technique called dry skin brushing is simple and effective. It increases circulation and stimulates the lymphatic system to eliminate toxins and excess water.

To dry brush your skin, you should use a natural fibre brush, not plastic or nylon. Use the following technique several times a week in the morning before you step into the shower or bath:

- Using circular or figure-eight motions, brush your skin lightly, starting with your torso and working toward your heart.
- Move to your legs, then your arms.
- Give special attention to your thighs, buttocks, and the backs of your arms and legs.
- Make sure to brush the palms of your hands and soles of your feet.
- Do not dry brush your face. Use a dry washcloth, instead.
- Be gentle and do not brush over any sore spots or open wounds.

On days when you have more time, give your body a salt scrub. This is an excellent whole-body treatment because the salts serve as both an exfoliant and a detoxifer. Salt scrub formulas can be purchased but are relatively inexpensive to make at home. Simply mix 25g (1oz) of ground sea salt with 10 to 12 drops of any stimulating essential oil to make a paste that you can spread easily over your body. To get a salt scrub with more 'feel', use ingredients common to the kitchen.

You will need ¼ cup Dead Sea salt, ¼ cup ground oats, ⅓ cup warmed virgin olive oil and 10 drops essential oils of your choice.

When using either scrub, rub small handfuls at a time over your entire body using small circular motions and following the recommendations above. Follow any whole-body scrub with a shower and an application of moisturizer.

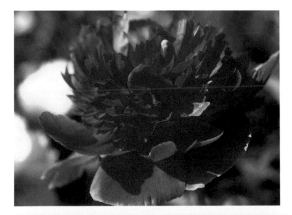

Give yourself a body wrap

Detoxifying herbal body wraps are popular at spas and are the ultimate in luxury. Wraps are especially good for drawing out nicotine and alcohol. They detoxify by increasing perspiration, encouraging circulation and promoting drainage of the lymphatic system. You can mimic a spa-quality herbal wrap in your home, though be warned: it can get messy, especially the preparation and clean-up afterwards. But at a fraction of the cost, it can be worth it.

Detoxifying herbs that can be part of a wrap include:

- Dandelion roots and leaves
- Echinacea root
- Garlic cloves (if you dare!)
- Parsley leaves
- Alfalfa leaves
- Comfrey roots and leaves
- Dried cascara sagrada

You will need the following:

- Three large handfuls of detoxifying herbs
- A large super-clean bucket or utility tub
- Two very large, soft towels, such as beach towels
- A plastic sheet longer and wider than you are
- A clean tile, wood or linoleum floor on which to lay out the plastic

Put the herbs in the bucket and fill it with very hot water. Wait a few minutes, then submerge the towels in the water. Let everything steep for 5 to 10 minutes. Remove the towels and squeeze them gently. (The idea is to leave as much water in as possible but not have them dripping.) Remove your clothes and wrap the towels tightly around you. Remember, you must work quickly! The hotter the towels, the better the results. Lie down on the plastic and relax. Stay put for at least 15 minutes, then unwrap yourself slowly.

Body wraps are not intended to be a quick weight-loss device. Make sure to replace the fluid lost by drinking 8 to 10 glasses of mineral water over the next 24 hours. Also, skip refined sugars and foods and eat organic fruits and vegetables.

HOW TO MAKE AROMATIC WATER

Misting your face with clean, fresh water during your spa treatment is nice, but misting your face with floral water is even nicer.

To make floral water, take 3 handfuls of petals from your favourite aromatic flower, put them in a large pot, and cover the petals completely with water. Heat the flowers and water over low heat and simmer until the water reduces by half. After the water cools, strain it into a clean, 350ml (12fl oz) mist bottle. Gently squeeze water from the petals until the bottle is full.

If the water comes out tinted, it may stain your skin. Either use fewer flowers or choose another flower that doesn't discolour the water.

Caution If you have hay fever or skin allergies, you should test whether you are allergic to a flower before using it. Rub some petals on a small area of skin and leave it for 48 hours. If any irritation develops, don't use the flower in your bathwater or on your face.

You can do a less-messy detoxifying body wrap by using essential oils. Mix 5 drops each of cypress, lemon and juniper oils, plus 1 teaspoon of sea salt in a 350ml (12fl oz) bottle of hot mineral water. Then simply spray the hot, wet towels before applying.

Keeping your make-up pure

When it comes to chemically produced, commercial personal care products, cosmetics rank as the most toxic.

Look at the labels of the products you are using. If the ingredients list looks like a jumble of letters with suffixes such as 'ben', 'ply' and 'thyl', then you know the cosmetics you are using are not all-natural. Even water-based products such as lotions, shampoos, conditioners, shower gels and bubble baths contain chemicals. That's because water must be preserved in order to give the products a shelf life. (Remember, water is a favourite gathering place for mould and fungus.)

Anything that has 'petro', 'lum' or anything that sounds like petroleum-in-hiding is exactly that. Mineral oil, which is commonly found in cosmetics, is a petroleum derivative.

Skin keeps its softness and texture as a result of naturally occurring triglycerides, wax esters, fatty acids and vitamin E. As chemicals, pollution and the sun sap the skin of these natural oils, they need to be replaced. Look for products that claim to contain such things as avocado oil, clove oil or any fruit or vegetable oil.

Cleanse twice a day A morning-and-night cleansing routine is important, especially if you live in a big city where environmental pollution from things like car exhaust, diesel fumes and chemical plants is high. Good cleansing is important even if you don't wear makeup.

Do not use soap and water to clean your face Rather, use a mild, soap-free moisturizing cleanser that's right for your skin type. Ingredients that are particularly good for your skin include aloe vera, lanolin, olive oil, orange oil, sweet almond oil, vitamin C and vitamin E.

Shed dead skin Exfoliating tender facial skin requires a tactic that differs from the whole-body brushing routine described earlier. In addition to getting rid of dead skin, exfoliating helps to get dirt and makeup out of your pores, preventing them from clogging and allowing them to accept nutrients. Exfoliate once a day, at night. Natural ingredients in exfoliants include such things as ground oats, ground almonds or spices and natural plant oils such as almond, olive and orange.

Give skin a daily tone Applying a fresh, soothing toning lotion goes beyond making your skin feel refreshed; it decongests pores and equalizes the skin's pH. It also removes any traces of dirt still left on your face. Use a low-alcohol or an alcohol-free toner.

Moisturize Moisturizers help to feed the skin with important nutrients and help to protect the skin from harsh elements. Depending on your skin type, you should moisturize day and night. Look for ingredients such as glycerin, vitamin C, borage oil, blackcurrant oil, rice bran oil and those that offer sun protection.

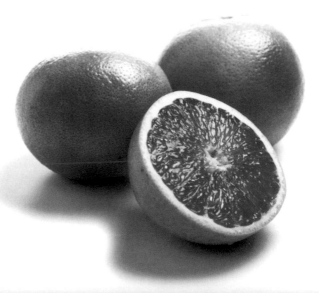

Chapter 13
Targeted plans
For specific conditions

Toxicity affects us in hundreds of ways. Even though some detox remedies are used across the board to address a number of health concerns, many others are best used in a tailored approach to specific conditions.

In this chapter you'll find detox strategies for some of the most common health threats – conditions that can damage your health and perniciously erode your energy, motivation and physical and emotional strength. It's always a good idea to work with a health care practitioner who combines detox procedures with mainstream medicine, but the plans have been designed with safety in mind. You can do them yourself at home, without spending a fortune on expensive procedures. Start now and feel the difference.

If you have a particular condition that's challenging you, you'll find a range of practical tips and techniques that will help your body to use the power of detoxification to ameliorate the problem. Remember, though, that curing a single condition wins a battle. If you want to win the war – returning your body to vibrant health – you'll still need the essentials of purification detailed in the other sections of this book.

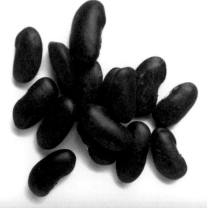

Ageing

Stay younger for longer
Every year, people are living just a little bit longer. This is partly due to our successes in battling diseases, but it's also because scientists are unlocking the secrets of ageing itself.

Cells in your body divide a certain number of times, then die and are replaced by new cells. This process slows with age, however. Muscles get less flexible, bones weaken, immunity declines and your organs get tired. Some of these changes are inevitable, but new research suggests that it may be possible to put the brakes on our own declines.

Your detox plan

Strategy 1: Eliminate pollutants
Over a lifetime, the liver, intestines and other organs work overtime to eliminate pollutants from the body, and all that extra effort accelerates the ageing process.

A healthy diet and regular exercise are essential steps in any detoxification plan. At the same time, you need to cleanse your body of disease-causing chemical wastes.

Eat more beans They contain phytates, which bind to toxins in the intestine and eliminate them from the body. Ideally, you should be eating beans a few times a week.

Scientists have known for a long time that when animals are given about one-third fewer calories than normal, their life expectancy jumps by about one-third. If the same were true in humans, cutting about 600 calories out of your daily diet would increase your life expectancy from the current eighty three years (for women) to an average of one hundred years.

Consider life in Okinawa, Japan, where a low-calorie diet is typical – and where people are 40 times more likely than people in other parts of the world to celebrate their 100th birthdays. No one knows for sure why reducing calories increases longevity, although it may be linked to accompanying reductions in insulin levels. Calorie restriction seems to be the only proven way to extend life. Keep in mind, though, that cutting calories to this extent basically means that you will be going hungry all the time. This can be hard and few of us have the stamina, or desire, to live that way. But eating less is certainly healthier in the long run. If most of us followed this simple rule, we'd live longer, be healthier and feel younger.

Protect your liver with milk thistle Milk thistle contains a chemical compound, silymarin, that enhances the liver's production of glutathione, a chemical toxin neutralizer, by 35 percent. It also helps damaged liver cells to regenerate. The recommended dose is 200mg three times daily.

Drink a lot of water You need at least eight glasses a day, because water dilutes chemical concentrations in the blood and helps all the organs of elimination to work more efficiently.

Keep the colon clean Toxins accumulate in the stools, and if you don't have daily bowel movements, many of these toxins seep back into your bloodstream. A high-fibre diet is the most efficient way to keep stools moving. Eat plenty of fruits and vegetables and have modified fasts, eating only raw foods and fresh vegetables, several times a year.

Give yourself plenty of downtime Uncontrolled stress lowers immunity, increases blood pressure in some cases, and can make you look and feel older than your years. The more you relax, the more efficiently your liver and other organs will be able to detoxify your body.

Strategy 2: Block damage to cells

Many age-related diseases are caused, in part, by free radicals. You can fight them by increasing your dietary intake of antioxidant nutrients that bind to tissue-damaging molecules and block their harmful effects. These are the antioxidants that experts recommend most.

Vitamin E It blocks free-radical damage in the fatty membranes that surround cells, and it appears to counteract some of the negative effects of air pollution, heavy metals and other environmental toxins. Vitamin E also improves immunity and may reduce the risk of age-related diseases, including heart disease and some cancers.

You need 150 IU of vitamin E daily for its anti-ageing effects. It's hard to get that amount from diet alone, so take a daily supplement, and increase your intake of vitamin E–rich foods, such as nuts, seeds and wheat germ.

Selenium A mineral that works together with vitamin E to reduce cell irritation, it binds to harmful toxins such as mercury, arsenic and cadmium and reduces their destructive effects in the body. Also, selenium is a powerful antioxidant that strengthens the ability of the immune system to seek out and destroy cancerous cells. Selenium can be toxic in amounts greater than 900mcg, and it's not wise to take more than 200mcg per day.

Carotenoids Deep green and bright orange fruits and vegetables are rich in carotenoids – extremely powerful antioxidants that reduce damage to cellular DNA that sets the stage for cancer and other degenerative diseases, such as eye diseases.

Vitamin C In addition to being a strong antioxidant, vitamin C prevents the conversion of nitrites, chemicals in meats and many other foods, into carcinogenic nitrosamines. Vitamin C also reduces irritation from air pollution and passive smoking. Try to get at least 200 to 500mg daily.

L-cysteine It's a sulphur-containing amino acid that neutralizes free radicals and helps the liver produce glutathione, one of the most potent antioxidants. Food sources of L-cysteine include avocados, grapefruit and tomatoes.

B vitamins Many older adults have difficulty absorbing B vitamins, which strengthen nerve coatings and improve memory. The B vitamins are essential nutrients in any detox plan because they help the body to eliminate homocysteine, an amino acid-like compound that increases the risk of heart disease. To lower homocysteine levels and make improvements in brain function, take 10mg of B_6, 1,000mcg of B_{12} and 1mg of folic acid.

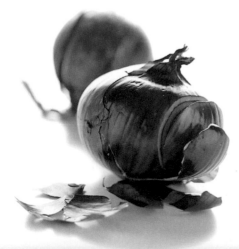

Allergies & asthma

Better breathing
Exposure to allergens such as pollens can unleash a flood of histamine, leukotrienes and other inflammatory compounds in the body. Asthma is a bit more complicated, but the results are similar: exposure to allergens or even a breath of cold air can cause tiny airways in the lungs to get constricted and inflamed.

Besides avoiding these problematic substances, you also need to restore the strength of your body's protective barriers.

Your detox plan

Strategy 1: Cleanse your body's filters
Here's what doctors advise you do to boost your body's natural defences.

Clean out fast You need to lower the burden on the immune system so that it copes with airborne irritants more appropriately. A two-day water or juice fast is one of the quickest and safest ways to remove toxins from the colon and promote better digestion. At the very least, eat a lot more fruit, vegetables and legumes.

Watch out for additives Many people with asthma and allergies are sensitive to food additives and preservatives, including sulphites, tartrazine and sodium benzoate. Always eat organic foods and drink purified water.

Exercise often Regular exercise improves the ability of the lungs to take in oxygen and dispel carbon dioxide. It helps the lungs, liver and kidneys to excrete toxins more efficiently. It also makes you sweat, and perspiration carries toxins out of the body through the skin. However, if your asthma is exercise-induced, take medical advice before undertaking new exercises.

Strategy 2: Control your diet

Allergies and asthma can be managed with some easy yet effective changes to your diet and lifestyle.

Have a little red Red wine contains flavonoids and a little may help asthma sufferers.

Shake the salt A diet high in sodium may make bronchioles, tiny airways in the lungs, more sensitive to histamine. Read labels and buy low or no-sodium foods, and use less salt.

Have a cup of tea Tea, apples and onions are excellent sources of quercetin, an antioxidant that inhibits the release of histamine and also tames free radicals, so increase your intake of these three foods. Cut down on sugar in your tea, though.

Cut animal foods A diet high in meats or dairy foods can trigger more asthma attacks. But the omega-3 fats found in fish oils are good for you.

Strategy 3: Reduce allergens

The combination of environmental toxins and less-than-perfect diets can cause junctions between cells in the intestine walls to become 'leaky' and allow undigested food particles to pass into the bloodstream. The immune system reacts to these particles, potentially making you more vulnerable to allergies.

Cut out dietary culprits Keep track of everything you eat for a month or two. When you have an allergy or asthma flare-up, check your notes to see which foods you ate prior to the symptoms occurring. Then eliminate those foods, one at a time, for three to four weeks to see if it makes a difference.

Rotate your diet Don't eat any one food more often than once every three or four days. Giving yourself a few days' break from specific foods can reduce allergy flare-ups and also reduce the risk of developing new allergies in the future.

Strategy 4: Wash out inflammation

Histamine and other chemicals produced by the immune system cause an inflammatory response in the respiratory system. To reduce inflammation:

Increase vitamin C Take 500 to 1,000mg of vitamin C daily. It blocks the effects of free radicals and appears to prevent asthma attacks by making the airways less likely to go into spasm.

Eat more tomatoes Lycopene, an antioxidant found in tomatoes, and present particularly in canned tomatoes, can reduce asthma symptoms.

Strategy 5: Clear out congestion

Try some natural steps to help mucus flow more easily and to cleanse your body of congestion-causing chemicals.

Avoid milk, and drink a lot of water Dairy foods may trigger congestion. So go easy on milk, and drink plenty of water. It makes mucus thinner so that it drains out of the body rather than accumulating in the respiratory tract.

Get rid of excess phlegm Breathing hot, moist air can help to eliminate mucus from your airways and make breathing easier. Another option during allergy season is sinus irrigation, with a neti pot. See 'How to use a neti pot' on page 62.

Arthritis

Calming inflammation

If you have arthritis, the body's immune system pours powerful cells and chemicals onto the site of the problem – your knees or hips, for example – but at the same time those chemicals damage the tissue they're meant to repair.

There are more than 100 forms of arthritis, the most common being osteoarthritis and rheumatoid arthritis.

Since rheumatoid arthritis is triggered by a misbehaving immune system, and the immune system is affected by what you eat, it makes sense that changes in your diet can make a real difference. Osteoarthritis is caused by mechanical problems in the joints rather than a whole-body immune response.

Your detox plan

Strategy 1: Turn off immune response triggers

The most important strategy is to eliminate toxins that can stimulate your immune system to launch its misguided attacks.

Cut back on meat protein In people who are sensitive to them, the fats in animal products can switch on the body's production of inflammation-causing chemicals called prostaglandins.

The secret to detoxifying the body is to eat a diet that consists entirely of all-natural foods with very high nutritional content that are free of preservatives, salt or sugar.

Take fish oil supplements In high doses – usually about 9g to 12g (approx. ⅓oz) a day – fish oil can reduce joint inflammation and cut pain.

Track and eliminate Many people with arthritis are sensitive to specific foods. Keep a food diary for a few months. At the same time, jot down when you have arthritis flare-ups. Comparing the two lists will give you an idea of what foods are most likely to cause problems.

Strategy 2: Stop the pain with vitamins and supplements

The trick to quelling arthritis pain is to lower levels of pain-causing prostaglandins and substance P, a chemical messenger than carries pain signals from the painful area to the brain. Take steps to flush your joints of waste products from your body's normal metabolism.

Clear out wastes with vitamin C Vitamin C helps to fight free radicals and may relieve joint pain.

Take a pineapple pill Supplements that contain bromelain, a chemical compound extracted from pineapples, lower levels of inflammation.

Block out substance P The next time you have an arthritis flare-up, apply capsaicin cream, available over the counter, to the sore area. It works by counter-stimulation and counteracts the pain impulses of arthritis.

Strategy 3: Employ nature's pharmacy

Some natural healers include the following in a plan intended to lessen the effects of arthritis.

Turmeric It contains chemical compounds that lower levels of prostaglandins and other inflammatory substances. You can include turmeric in food, or you can buy it in the form of an herbal supplement.

Ginger. Eating 1 to 3 teaspoons of ginger daily gives significant relief from pain and swelling. You can enjoy ginger as a spice, drink it as a tea, or take it as a supplement.

Willow bark Made into a tea, willow bark delivers high levels of salicin, an aspirin-like chemical that lowers levels of inflammatory prostaglandins.

Nettles Eaten as a vegetable, an average serving of cooked stinging nettle provides more than 3mg of boron, a mineral that is recommended for both rheumatoid arthritis and osteoarthritis. All you have to do is simmer the nettle leaves in water for 5 to 10 minutes, or until tender.

Good bacteria Probiotic supplements contain live, beneficial bacteria that take up

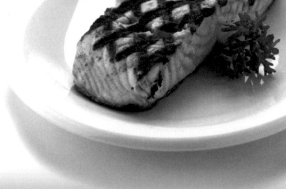

residence in the intestine and crowd out less healthy bacteria. Bacterial toxins can be related to rheumatoid arthritis, and you can reduce their levels with probiotics.

Strategy 4: Fasting to speed recovery

If joint pains are triggered by foods, fasting for several days gives the entire body a chance to recover. Drink fruit juices, vegetable juices or herbal teas during your fast. A modified fast can usually help to ease arthritis pain while providing your body with nutrients. Obviously, you don't want to fast for extended periods on your own. To be safe, check with your doctor before you try fasting for any longer than a day.

For more information on safe and healthy fasting, see Chapter 6.

Strategy 5: Eat well and lose weight

People who are overweight tend to suffer more pain from osteoarthritis because they carry a heavier load, and the extra pressure on their joints invariably causes more pain. Studies suggest that people who lose as little as 4.5 to 7kg (10–15lb) often feel a dramatic reduction in soreness.

It's a good idea to cut back on fats when you're trying to lose weight, but there is one type you'll want to include in an anti-arthritis diet: the omega-3 fatty acids, found primarily in cold-water fish (such as mackerel, trout and salmon). These fatty acids reduce levels of prostaglandins and leukotrienes, both of which contribute to inflammation. Two to three weekly servings is probably enough.

Binges

Too much food or drink

Here are some cleansing steps to help you to start getting your cravings for food and drink under control and reducing the harm that they can do to your body over time.

Your detox plan

Strategy 1: Shake the sugar

Banish sugar from your life Sugar is almost like a drug in its addictiveness. Once you give it up, the cravings usually end in one to three weeks.

Give up coffee for a few weeks Along with colas and other caffeinated beverages, coffee can produce intense sugar cravings.

Mop up the excess The level of glucose (sugar) in your blood rises sharply when you overdo it. The pancreas releases insulin to bring glucose back down, but sometimes it overshoots. When that happens, your blood sugar levels plummet and you crave food to restore a kind of balance. The minerals chromium and magnesium can help because they stabilize blood sugar and keep cravings under control. You may want to supplement with 200mcg of chromium and 500 to 700mg of magnesium daily. You can divide each supplement into two doses. Take one in the late morning and another in the afternoon (times when blood sugar starts to slump). You'll still need to restrict your intake of dietary sugar, but the minerals will help to keep cravings under control.

Strategy 2: Turn off the triggers

Here are a few ways to put yourself back in control of your cravings.

Calm cravings with zinc This mineral derails out-of-control cravings by activating a brain chemical that sends 'stop eating' signals to the brain. Get at least 15mg daily – the amount found in most multivitamin supplements.

Clear out depression's cobwebs Since nearly everyone who suffers from food cravings has some degree of depression, you'll want to take steps to clear it out of your life.

- **Start with 5-HTP** Your brain converts this supplement into serotonin, a chemical that improves mood and curbs appetite. Take 50mg of 5-HTP three times daily for six weeks.

If you don't notice a reduction in cravings, increase the dose to 100mg. If you're on other antidepressants, check with your doctor before supplementing with 5-HTP. Bananas may prove helpful, instead.

- **Take St. John's wort** This over-the-counter supplement is just as effective as prescription drugs for treating mild to moderate depression. It improves mood, stabilizes appetite and makes it easier for the brain to send stop-eating signals when you're full. Take 300mg two or three times daily. As with 5-HTP, don't combine it with antidepressants without checking with your doctor. **Caution:** people taking the contraceptive pill, warfarin and cyclosporin – as well as certain other classes of drug – should not take St John's wort as it lowers blood levels.

Drink plenty of water Your body often confuses dehydration with hunger. Try drinking two glasses of water, preferably with a squeeze of lemon. Wait a few minutes. You'll probably find that your craving has gone.

Strategy 3: Head-off hangovers

Moderate drinking (up to one drink daily for women and two for men) protects against heart disease and can help to lower blood pressure and the risk of stroke. Drinking too much, however, has the opposite effect and can devastate your personal life along with your health.

Your body's detoxification systems need to work in order to clean alcohol from your blood. You'll feel a lot better when you cleanse your body of alcohol-related toxins and waste products.

If you must drink, think 'light' Darker, sweeter drinks, such as red wine and whisky, contain more cogeners – (organic molecules such as methanol that increase the head-pounding effects) than lighter drinks such as white wine or vodka.

Eliminate acetaldehyde accumulation If you experience hangovers even after modest drinking, it's possible that one of your liver's detoxification

pathways is more sluggish than it should be. This can lead to buildups of acetaldehyde, a toxic substance that causes morning-after discomfort. To cleanse the liver:

- **Take a B-complex supplement** It helps the liver to cleanse itself more quickly
- **Mix a little lemon juice** and a teaspoonful of cayenne pepper in a tablespoon of olive oil, and take it once or twice when you're suffering the next-day blues. Don't take any more than a few tablespoonfuls of olive oil. Too much can cause the gallbladder to go into spasms.
- **Sip dandelion tea** It is among the best liver remedies and helps with cellular repair after exposure to cell-damaging toxins. Dandelion is a mild diuretic, so make sure you drink extra water when taking it. This herbal tea is available in convenient tea bags.
- **Take milk thistle** This supplement contains a chemical compound, silymarin, that stimulates liver cells and helps them to rid the body of alcohol-related waste products.

Drink more water When you have a hangover, you need to drink water to counter dehydration, so take in as much as you can. Water dilutes toxins and waste products and also reverses dehydration, the main cause of alcohol-related discomfort.

Increase fibre High-fibre foods can make a difference when you've had too much to drink. Fibre sops up alcohol and alcohol by-products in the intestine and speedily carries them out of the body in the stool.

Tropical stomach soother Have a few slices of papaya or a fruit smoothie with papaya. It contains papain and protease enzymes that make proteins easier to digest and soothes an upset stomach.

Blood cleansing

Healthy blood for healthy cells

Every organ in your body, every cell and artery and bit of tissue, is linked by blood. The heart sends blood through your system, delivering oxygen and nutrients and carting away wastes. But blood also carries toxins that can damage your health. We inadvertently flood our systems with synthetic, disease-causing toxins that weaken the body's ability to keep itself clean.

The way to cleanse the blood is to ensure that all of the organs of elimination are working well. Here's a set of strategies to detoxify the blood and ensure that it can transport materials for health rather damaging toxins.

Your detox plan

Strategy 1: Cleanse your liver
The liver has a remarkable ability to regenerate itself but of course it will perform better with periodic cleansing.

Drink dandelion root tea It enhances the flow of blood to the liver. It's especially important if you're taking antidepressants, which impede the liver's detoxification pathways. Drink several cups daily.

Start the day with fibre Sprinkle a tablespoonful of psyllium seeds or oat bran on your morning cereal. Eat more fruits, vegetables, legumes and whole grains.

Drink plenty of water – at least eight glasses daily. It reduces the body's concentration of toxins and makes it easier for the liver, kidneys and other elimination organs to clear them from the blood.

Strategy 2: Cleanse your lungs
Your lungs remove toxic wastes, including carbon dioxide, that are produced by your body's normal metabolism and carried in your blood.

Exercise daily because anything that increases your normal rate of respiration enhances the ability of hairlike filters in your lungs to carry out waste products along with any build-up of mucus. Exercise also increases the replacement of carbon dioxide and other waste gases in your blood with energizing oxygen.

Strategy 3: Cleanse your skin
Ensuring that your skin works at peak condition helps to clear toxins from your blood.

Dry brush daily Use a soft brush to rub every inch of your skin, always brushing toward the centre of your body. The best time to do this is right before you take a shower.

Scrub with salt Health food shops sell a variety of salt scrubs, stimulating salts that increase metabolism and speed the elimination of toxins when you rub them on your body. The salts also act like dry brushing and increase lymph drainage.

Soak in Epsom salts Adding Epsom salts (magnesium sulphate) to the bath is particularly helpful because it pulls toxins out of the skin.

Follow hot with cold One of the best ways to encourage the detoxification of your skin and lymphatic system is to follow a hot bath or shower with a cool rinse, and repeat the process at least three times.

Strategy 4: Cleanse your kidneys
These organs filter blood and remove urea, salts, excess minerals and other potentially toxic wastes from your blood. Every drop of your blood passes

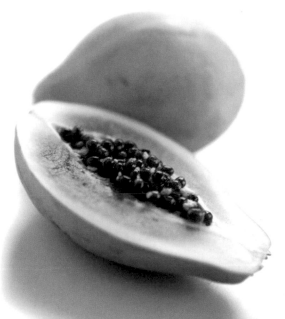

through your kidneys about 20 times an hour. It's possible for your kidneys to get congested with wastes, work more slowly and allow more impurities to stay in your bloodstream. Here's what you need to do to keep them clean.

Reach for the water bottle Drink at least 2 litres (3½ pints) of water a day, or more if you're bigger than average, live in a hot climate or exercise a lot.

Switch to dandelion leaf tea Dandelion leaf tea has a diuretic effect and is also an excellent source of potassium. That's important because most prescription diuretics remove potassium from the body. Dandelion will help to keep the balance.

Strategy 5: Cleanse your colon

Many toxins are eliminated in the stools, but some are reabsorbed back into the bloodstream, especially if you are constipated. Cleaning your colon regularly will help to ensure that toxins leave your body when stools do.

Fast regularly It's the most effective tool for detoxifying the colon. It reduces the body's toxic burden and can help relieve arthritis, eczema and many other common conditions. We talk about fasting in detail in Chapter 6.

Consider a colonic procedure For advice on self-administered enemas and colonic irrigation during a fast, see 'Flushing the toxic colon' on page 60 and also pages 21 and 72.

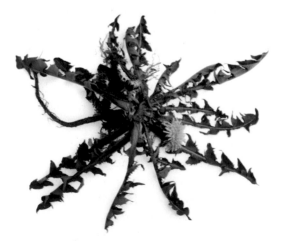

Cancer prevention

Keep your cells healthy

Most body cells are continuously being renewed. If a cell is damaged during the division process – as a result of exposure to harmful, toxic substances in the body – it can spin out of control. The result is cancer-cell growth and multiplication that can't be stopped.

Your body is equipped to eliminate or neutralize toxins in the colon, kidneys, liver and other organs. But our modern world is so full of toxins that the body can't always cope. Air pollution, industrial chemicals, pesticides and even chemicals or hormones in the body can disrupt the cellular machinery and trigger cancer growth.

Try to avoid pollutants whenever possible and to minimize pollutants in the body with the following detoxification plan.

Your detox plan

Strategy 1: Control your hormones

Two of the hormones that play key roles in determining who we are – oestrogen in women and testosterone in men – are also the ones that often promote tumour growth. You obviously wouldn't want to eliminate these hormones, but it's essential to take steps to minimize their potentially harmful effects.

Say yes to soya Tofu, tempeh and other soya foods are rich in plant chemicals called isoflavones, which reduce the impact of oestrogen in the body cells and possibly reduce a woman's breast cancer risk. A soya-rich diet is good for men, as well, possibly because these foods lessen the effect of oestrogen, which men also have and which encourages protate cancers to grow.

Add tofu to your next stir-fry, steam some fresh soyabeans, or munch on soya nuts and snacks. Switch from cow's milk to soya milk. Try grilling your steaks with soya sauce and a hint of garlic.

Trim your risk with fibre The less a woman is exposed to her own reproductive hormones, the lower her risk of developing breast cancer. A fibre-rich diet of fruits, vegetables, whole grains and legumes lowers levels of oestrone, a type of oestrogen associated with higher rates of cancer. Fibre also helps to flush toxins from the colon, so consider adding a fibre supplement to your diet.

Lose weight, lower your risk After the menopause, much of the body's oestrogen is produced by fatty tissues, and much of the body's overload of toxins is stored in fatty tissues. Women who maintain a healthy weight or who successfully lose weight by exercising regularly and eating well, have lower levels of toxins and oestrogen and seem less likely to get breast cancer than overweight women.

Strategy 2: Eliminate toxins

We live in a remarkably toxic environment, and your body's cells pay the price. Take advantage of proven body cleansers that seek out potential carcinogens and carry them out of the body.

Load up on citrus Lemons, limes and oranges contain limonene which stimulates the ability of the immune system to destroy cancer cells before they can multiply. Citrus fruits also contain glucarase, a compound that neutralizes carcinogens and rushes them out of the body. Choose orange juice for your breakfast drink.

Eat dandelion salad Or drink dandelion tea. It helps the liver to eliminate and break down toxins before they have a chance to damage cells. It helps the liver to detoxify the body.

Cut carcinogens with crucifers Broccoli, brussels sprouts, cabbage and other crucifers are rich in sulphoraphane, a chemical compound that increases the body's output of cancer-fighting enzymes. Crucifers convert oestrogen into a form that's less likely to trigger cell changes that can lead to cancer.

Detoxify with garlic Eat a lot of it. It's one of the most potent cancer-fighting herbs as it contains chemicals that boost the production of enzymes that detoxify potential carcinogens. Substances in garlic may also slow the growth of breast, skin and colon cancers. Other chemicals in garlic help the body to excrete carcinogenic toxins.

Cut the saturated fat A high-fat diet increases levels of cell-damaging molecules, increases production of testosterone and oestrogen, and steps up the body's production of bile acid, which may be transformed into cancer-causing compounds. A diet low in saturated fat can also reduce your risk of colon and prostate cancers. People who eat less fat usually eat more plant foods. The fibre in these foods helps to trap cancer-causing substances in the colon and rushes them out of the body before they can trigger dangerous cell changes.

Strategy 3: Build your immune system

Detoxify with antioxidants Every day your body's cells are damaged by free radicals that strip away electrons and set the stage for cancer-causing mutations. It's essential to load up on foods that contain the 'big three' antioxidants – beta-carotene and vitamins C and E. They reduce the harmful effects of free radicals and protect cells from life-threatening changes.

- *Beta-carotene*, in sweet potatoes, spinach and other richly coloured vegetables, stimulates the release of immune cells that hunt down and destroy cancer cells. The recommended dosage is no more than 7mg a day – although it may be safer to try to get this through diet rather than supplements.

- *Vitamin C*, in addition to being one of the most powerful antioxidants, has been shown to prevent carcinogenic compounds from forming in the digestive tract. Try 500 to 1,000mg per day. If you have any digestive problems with vitamin C, lower the dose until symptoms go.

- **Vitamin E** also stimulates the immune system's fight against cancer cells and blocks the effects of free radicals in the body's fatty tissues. Since it's difficult to get enough vitamin E from food, consider taking 150 IUs in supplement form.

Colds

Just say 'Go!' to viruses

When a virus infects a small patch of cells lining the nose, the immune system pushes out a host of chemicals known as inflammatory mediators that cause blood vessels to leak and dilate, stimulate pain nerve fibres and turn on the mucus.

The virus will eventually get mopped up by your immune system, but you'll keep having symptoms unless you find some way to cleanse your body of all the chemicals that make you feel so bad.

Your detox plan

Strategy 1: Evict the virus

Scientists have tried for years to find a cure for the common cold, and they're still trying. The good news is that some of the same foods and herbs that cleanse your body and reduce symptoms will also prevent these miserable infections from taking hold in the first place.

Reach for herbal remedies Both goldenseal and echinacea have been shown to help to relieve colds in some studies, but not all. Both are readily available in convenient capsules or tinctures.

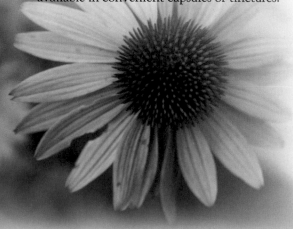

Sip ginger tea Studies have shown that ginger contains chemical compounds called sesquiterpenes, which help to suppress rhinoviruses, the most common family of cold viruses. Other compounds in ginger, gingerols and shogaols, reduce pain, fever and coughing.

To make ginger tea, add about ½ teaspoon each of ginger powder, cinnamon and fennel seeds to a cup of hot water. Let the tea steep for about 10 minutes, strain out the herbs and drink it while it's hot. You can also buy tea bags that contain ginger and other spices. Drink several cups a day for the duration of the cold.

Load up on fruit and vegetables Many fruits and vegetables contain glutathione, a chemical compound that stimulates the release of your body's own immune cells that mop up viruses for disposal. In addition, fruits and vegetables contain a variety of antioxidants that knock out free radicals, which are produced in abundance when you have a cold.

Feed a cold Dutch scientists report that eating causes an increase in gamma interferon, an immune chemical that stimulates the body's ability to destroy and clear itself of cold viruses.

Strategy 2: Clear out congestion

The mucus that forms in your throat and nose is a trap for toxins, so try some of these tips that also help you to breathe more easily and sleep more comfortably.

Press away congestion Firmly pressing the web of skin between your thumb and index finger for about a minute will help break up congestion and remove mucus from your body. You can use the same acupressure technique on the upper ridges of your eye sockets close to the bridge of your nose, or just to the sides of your nostrils along your smile line.

Mop up with vitamin C Vitamin C can help to reduce stuffiness and congestion and also knocks down levels of free radicals.

Drink pineapple juice Fresh pineapple juice is loaded with vitamin C and also helps the body to break down mucus and expel it from the body. Drink 100ml to175ml (3½–6fl oz) of juice (diluted half-and-half with water) at least four times daily when you're battling a cold. Drink a variety of fruit and vegetable juices or use your blender to whip up a smoothie that includes fresh pineapple chunks.

Get hydrated Drink as much water as you can hold. Colds cause the body to lose tremendous amounts of fluids. Drinking lots of water will help to reduce throat scratchiness and headache, while at the same time making mucus thinner and easier to eliminate from the body.

Add some cayenne to your soup Along with other hot peppers, cayenne is rich in capsaicin, a fiery chemical that will make your nose run almost immediately after you ingest it, a sign that your body is overcoming the head-stuffing congestion.

Steam away congestion Breathing hot, moisture-laden air is among the best ways to liquefy mucus so that it drains from your nose and airways. Less congestion means less coughing, stuffiness and chest pain.

Strategy 3: Invigorate your body

When you're battling a cold, your purifying plan should include techniques that have been shown to stoke your body's immune response.

Run hot and cold Following a warm bath with a quick rinse in cold water constricts blood vessels and reduces fever and inflammation.

Free yourself from stress It doesn't matter whether you breathe deeply for a few minutes, do yoga for half an hour or simply take a quick walk around the block, as long as you manage to reduce anxiety and stress.

Strategy 4: Eliminate irritants

Take special care of your respiratory system when you are suffering from a cold. Air pollution also causes cells to dump into your body inflammatory chemicals that make your eyes puffy, your nose run and your eyes water. You can't avoid all air pollution, of course, but avoid smoky places and rush-hour traffic.

Digestion

Detox your digestive tract

When you get overloaded with toxins, contaminants that may include lead, mercury and other dangerous metals, leak out of your digestive system and into your blood. They can damage cells, cause depression and fatigue and even shorten your life.

Your detox plan

Strategy 1: Fasting

Fasting is probably the best approach because it gives the digestive organs a chance to rest and recuperate, while at the same time it purges toxins from the intestine, liver and other parts of your body. (See Chapter 6 on fasting and cleansing.)

Strategy 2: Eat pure, feel pure

There are many ways to detoxify the digestive tract. But perhaps the most effective approach is to include in your diet easily digestible foods that have very specific (and quite different) toxin-fighting properties.

Recover from infections with B and C If you've recently had a cold or a bacterial infection, eat foods rich in B vitamins, such as whole grain bread, and foods with vitamin C, such as citrus, peppers and cabbage. Each of these nutrients helps to cleanse the body of toxins generated by harmful micro-organisms.

Scrub out additives with sulphur It's almost impossible to avoid food additives and preservatives that can drain your energy and weaken your health. So eat plenty of foods rich in sulphur, such as garlic, red peppers, egg yolks and

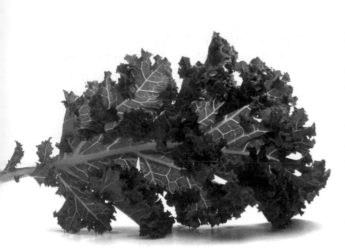

Milk thistle Studies show that this herb helps to neutralize a number of toxins. For more on Milk Thistle see pages 44–45.

Bentonite clay A purified clay that comes from volcanic ash and is very efficient at absorbing bacteria and contaminants and removing them from your body through the stool.

Flaxseed It acts as a gentle laxative and helps to eliminate toxins from the body. It's also an antioxidant that helps to neutralize the effects of free radicals.

Fatigue

Boost your energy

There are any number of herbs and supplements that can help to restore physical and mental energy, but they're much more effective when you first cleanse your body of the toxins that are dragging you down.

Your detox plan

Strategy 1: Reduce your toxic load

Toxicity occurs when your body accumulates more toxins and wastes than it can eliminate. Conversely, every cell and organ in your body works more efficiently when you help it to eliminate toxins. Here's what you need to do.

Start with a two-day liquid fast For two days, don't eat any food at all. Drink at least eight full glasses of water each day, more if you're still thirsty. See Chapter 6 for more about fasting. After the two-day fast, eat plenty of fresh fruits, vegetables and brown rice, and nothing else for five days. These easily digested foods will allow the intestine and liver to continue cleansing themselves.

Improve circulation with hydrotherapy This technique stimulates the pumping action of blood vessels and helps to flush out toxins, while at the same time bringing energizing oxygen to cells throughout your body. See page 22.

cruciferous vegetables. They help to eliminate food chemicals, in addition to many of the environmental pollutants that surround us.

Purify your gut with chlorophyll Found in green foods like cabbage, lettuce and parsley, chlorophyll cleanses the intestine, oxygenates the blood and speeds internal healing.

Give beneficial bacteria a home Live yogurt is among the healthiest foods you can eat. In addition to calcium and other nutrients, it contains probiotics, beneficial bacteria that take up residence in your intestine and help to displace harmful organisms.

Strategy 3: Supplement your detox diet

A healthy diet can do only so much to keep your system toxin-free. Fortunately, there are a number of over-the-counter supplements that break down toxins and help to eliminate them from your body. Use only one or two at a time.

Psyllium husk powder It absorbs water in the intestine and helps stools to pass through more quickly. This is important because stools are loaded with potential carcinogens and other toxins. The more quickly they move through your body, the less likely it is that the toxins they contain will leak through your intestinal wall and into your bloodstream.

Cleanse the intestine When you switch to easy-to-digest plant foods after the initial liquid fast, you'll naturally get a lot of fibre in your diet. Fibre accelerates the passage of stools and also binds to bile, a digestive fluid, in the intestine. The idea is to get bile moving out with the stools instead of hanging around waiting to be reabsorbed.

Get a lot of vitamin C Plan on taking 1,000mg three times a day for a week. It speeds the transit of stools and toxins out of the intestine, and it also detoxifies them so you're less likely to experience a 'healing crisis' during your fast.

Strategy 2: Stimulate your liver

The liver is the body's recycling plant for toxins, and it often gets overburdened and congested, which can lead to profound fatigue. There are several ways to stimulate the liver.

Eat fish several times a week Fish oils are essential for Phase 1 detoxification, the stage in which liver enzymes break down toxins. Eat fresh fish or you can take 2g daily of pharmaceutical-grade fish oil, which is guaranteed mercury-free.

Eat more fruits and vegetables They replenish your body's stores of glutathione, an amino acid that's essential for Phase 2 detox, which includes the breakdown of carcinogens as well as PCBs (a group of highly toxic chlorinated chemicals) and other industrial chemicals.

Eat high-quality proteins You get these from lean, organic meats, low-fat dairy products and eggs. They act on the liver's sulphation pathways, where industrial chemcials and bacterial toxins are broken down. Vegetable sources of sulphur include onions, celery, kale and soyabeans.

Get a handle on stress A flood of 'fight or flight' hormones such as cortisol make the body work overtime and block the liver's ability to detoxify chemical compounds.

Alternate-nostril breathing is a quick, efficient way to reduce mental and emotional stress. See page 79 for the method.

Strategy 3: Eat for energy

Eating the 'wrong' foods can leave you tired and drained. After you've cleansed your body of toxins, here's what you need to do to keep your energy levels high.

Avoid processed foods Even though food preservatives and additives are considered 'safe', over a lifetime, they dump a tremendous amount of chemicals into your body. These chemicals stress your liver and other elimination organs and wear you down.

Switch to decaf Caffeine is a diuretic that can dehydrate you. Dehydration increases the concentration of toxins that put extra strain on the liver and can slow your metabolism.

Take a pass on simple carbs Whole grains, legumes, fruits and vegetables are among the best foods you can eat because the complex carbohydrates they contain enter your body at a steady, energy-giving pace. Simple carbohydrates, on the other hand, send blood-sugar levels soaring. The body responds with a flood of insulin. Insulin quickly removes the sugars from the blood, and that's when your energy level drops into the basement.

Fertility

Increase your chances of conception

In both men and women, exposure to pesticides, industrial chemicals and other toxins has been linked to drops in fertility.

Your detox plan

Strategy 1: Reduce your exposure

You can't entirely avoid environmental chemicals, of course, but you can eliminate all or most of them from your body. One way to cut your risk of harmful exposure is to avoid using plastic water bottles, plastic food containers and plastic dishes to heat foods in the microwave. Many plastics contain oestrogen-like chemical compounds that leach into the body. Over time this may increase endometriosis in women and change the testosterone balance in men.

Strategy 2: Boost your body's natural cleaners

The more vitality you can bring to your skin and liver, the more your body will be able to rid itself of toxins you can't avoid. Here are some easy ways to accomplish that.

Work up a sweat The skin is one of the main organs of elimination. When you perspire from exercise or when you lounge in a dry or moist-heat sauna, toxins are released from fatty tissues and eliminated in perspiration.

Enjoy a very gentle massage Once every few days, have your partner stroke your skin with a feather light touch, moving from the outer parts of your body inward toward your heart. A 'soft' massage stimulates the lymph glands just beneath the skin and helps to accelerate the excretion of toxins that can interfere with fertility.

Drink marshmallow root tea It improves the ability of the digestive tract to process and eliminate wastes by its soothing effect, which also helps in the removal of phlegm from the respiratory tract.

Strategy 3: Improve your odds with nutrition

Dozens of physical problems can interfere with conception; for example, a man's sperm may become sluggish if he doesn't get a few key nutrients. A woman's body may be more receptive to pregnancy if she eats wholesome, organic foods. Both men and women can enhance their ability to eliminate toxins if they make a few simple dietary changes.

Load up on vitamin C The sperm in men who get adequate vitamin C tend to pick up speed and maintain their forward momentum. Vitamin C is a powerful antioxidant that helps to neutralize fertility-impairing free radicals. Take 250 to 1,000mg of vitamin C daily.

Get extra selenium and zinc Like vitamin C, this trace mineral is a powerful antioxidant that mops up free radicals from the body. Supplement your diet with about 200mcg of selenium daily.

It's also helpful to take a multivitamin supplement that includes zinc. It increases sperm levels, which is especially important for men who have been exposed to environmental chemicals.

Get the fat out of your diet High levels of dietary saturated fat can change your natural hormone balance. Fat increases levels of free radicals and inflammation. It also tends to raise levels of cholesterol, which clings to arteries and restricts bloodflow to the reproductive organs.

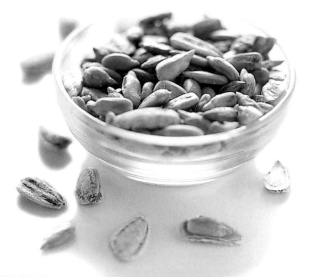

Shop from the fresh produce aisle A plant-based diet floods the body with phytochemicals, that block the harmful effects of toxic free radicals. Women who improve their diets and eat more plant foods and less meat tend to have lower levels of toxins and a lower incidence of endometriosis.

Flush toxins from the colon The liver, kidney, and other elimination organs are very efficient at removing toxins from your body. If you aren't having regular bowel movements, however, toxins that should be eliminated in the stools can be reabsorbed back into the blood. A high-fibre diet will help to clean out the colon. Good sources of fibre include beans, most fruit and vegetables and oatmeal.

Imbibe little or not at all Harvard researchers found that women who had more than one drink a day were 60 percent more likely to be infertile than women who abstained. Wine and other liquor can cause problems for men as well. Even small amounts of alcohol can lower testosterone and make sperm less hardy.

Cut the caffeine Scientists speculate that caffeine may alter a woman's hormone balance and interfere with her ability to ovulate.

Headaches & migraines

Banishing pain

Headaches may be common, but there's nothing normal about them. Something in your body is triggering the pain, causing a chemical cascade that irritates nerves, blood vessels, muscles or a combination of all three.

Impurities in the body can block the channels of circulation and prevent nutrients from effectively nourishing nerve tissue. This can also prevent waste products from being efficiently eliminated, allowing the buildup of toxins throughout your system. About 90 percent of headaches are the so-called tension-type.

Migraines are less common, but much more severe. They're probably triggered by the release of neuropeptides, substances that cause blood vessels to get dilated and inflamed.

Your detox plan: Headaches

Strategy 1: Clean out triggers

Since there are hundreds of potential pain triggers, your first step has to be to get them out of your life. Here's what you need to do.

Identify and eliminate key offenders Common culprits are chocolate, eggs, mustard, red wine, fermented foods, artificial sweeteners, sugar, dairy products, nuts or pickles. Eliminating some or most of these foods for a few weeks is a good way to test if they're a trigger for you. See page 28 for details of elimination diets.

Clear your home environment Make your home a safe haven by using air and water purifiers, along with non-toxic paints and cleaning agents.

Keep your blood sugar stable Sudden spikes and subsequent drops in blood sugar are a common cause of headaches. Eating small, frequent, nutritious meals will keep blood sugar more stable and keep headaches away.

Strategy 2: Sweep toxins from your body

You also need to purge your body of chemical build-ups that make you much more susceptible to headaches in the first place.

You can avoid some toxins by eating organic foods and avoiding products loaded with chemical dyes, preservatives and additives. But you do still have to support your body's natural detoxification pathways to give it the best possible chance.

Love the lowly dandelion Drink several cups of dandelion tea each day to increase blood-flow to your liver and help it to remove toxins. Other liver-protecting supplements include milk thistle and artichoke leaf.

Eat plenty of fibre Fresh fruits, whole grains, legumes and vegetables help your intestines to eliminate toxins more quickly.

Brush yourself Use a soft brush to dry rub your skin all over, always brushing toward the centre of your body. This helps to pump toxins out of your lymphatic system so that they can be processed by your liver and kidneys.

Warm up Relaxing in a warm environment opens blood vessels and helps your circulatory system to get rid of toxins. If you don't have access to a sauna, spend an occasional half-hour in a hot bath spiked with 2 cups of Epsom salts. See page 134 for more details.

Get professional care See a chiropractor, who can check your spine for misalignment. Back and neck problems may be the cause of headaches.

Strategy 3: Reduce muscle tension

Stress that causes muscles to bunch and tighten increases blood pressure and causes levels of pain-causing stress hormones to rise. Here are a few simple ways to relax.

Do yoga It's a great way to reduce emotional and physical stress Just about every health club offers yoga classes for every level of experience and physical fitness. Try some of the yoga exercises on pages 95–96.

Oil your temples Mix a few drops of lavender essential oil in a tablespoon of a carrier oil (such as olive or almond oil) and rub it on your temples. Lavender relaxes muscles and helps to reduce headache-causing stress.

Your detox plan: Migraines

Migraines affect less than 10 percent of people with headaches, but they cause a disproportionate amount of misery. Here are a few supplements that can make a real difference.

Try feverfew This head-protecting herb can be used to prevent migraines. It blocks the body's production of prostaglandins and other neurochemicals that cause inflammation and pain in blood vessels in the brain. Feverfew has to be taken regularly to be effective so don't try it only when you have a migraine.

Pump energy into your cells It's thought that abnormal functioning of mitochondria, the microscopic 'engines' that keep your cells running, may contribute to migraines. An over-the-counter supplement, coenzyme Q_{10}, seems to help mitochondria work more efficiently.

Heart disease

Clean your vessels, protect your heart

Nearly all of the major risk factors for heart disease can be reduced and often eliminated by following an action plan to scour your arteries and keep your body waste-free.

Your detox plan

Strategy 1: Tame toxic molecules

Your body produces antioxidants that stop some free-radical damage but not enough to stay entirely healthy, however.

That's why your body needs antioxidant-rich foods that contain substances that mop up free radicals and minimize their toxic effects. In addition to following a low-fat diet, rich in healthy grains and fresh produce, here are some other suggestions for you to consider.

Clean up with onions They're among the best sources of flavonoids, plant chemicals that are potent antioxidants. In addition to onions, other flavonoid-rich foods include apples, celery, berries, tea and red wine.

Avoid highly processed foods Most processed and preserved foods contain chemicals that turn into free radicals in the body. Try grilling or roasting some lean meat, chicken or fish, and enjoying it with a salad.

Scour your arteries with vitamin E This is probably the most important antioxidant for heart health because it prevents free radicals from damaging LDL, the harmful form of cholesterol. This is important because damaged LDL is more likely to cling to arteries, reduce bloodflow and set the stage for a future heart attack.

Vitamin E is found mainly in cooking oils and nuts. You may want to get extra amounts by taking a daily supplement that provides 150 IU.

Recycle E with C Vitamin C is a powerful antioxidant – one that also recharges vitamin E and keeps it active in the body.

Bet on beta-carotene It's a red-yellow plant pigment that turns into vitamin A in your body. At the same time, it mops up free radicals that can eventually damage your heart. The best food sources are dark green, leafy vegetables, such as spinach, and deep orange fruits and vegetables, such as sweet potatoes.

Strategy 2: Cut down the 'new risks'

Heart disease also strikes men and women who appear to do everything right. The reason is that many of us have chemicals in our bodies that greatly increase our risks. You can't eliminate these chemicals completely, but there are ways to knock them down to safer levels. Here's what doctors advise.

Fortify with fibre The 'roughage' in plant foods removes cholesterol from the body and lowers levels of a liver protein that's been linked to inflammation in the arteries. By promoting bowel function, it reduces the potential to reabsorb inflammatory chemicals from the intestine. You need about 25g (1oz) of fibre daily to protect your heart. Super sources include chickpeas, kidney beans, dried fruits and oatmeal.

Fight back with folate Folate is a B vitamin that lowers levels of homocysteine, an amino acid that can increase your risk of cardiovascular disease. Your doctor can check homocysteine levels with a simple blood test. If you have too much, make an extra effort to get plenty of folate and B vitamins in your diet. The best sources are green, leafy vegetables and fortified grains such as rice. You can also take a multivitamin supplement that provides 400mcg of folic acid daily.

Stop smoking to lower fibrinogen It's a blood protein that increases your tendency to form clots in your arteries.

Strategy 3: Muster your defences

Heart disease doesn't happen all at once. It's a decades-long process caused by ongoing assaults on the arteries. It's essential to cleanse your body of substances that put unnecessary stress on your system. Here's where to start.

Restrict sodium to lower blood pressure Hypertension (high blood pressure) is a complicated disease with dozens of possible treatment options, but everyone should make an effort to get no more than 2,000mg of sodium daily. Less than 1,500mg is even better. (One teaspoon of table salt contains approximately 2,000mg of sodium.)

Douse inflammation with fish People who eat several weekly servings of fish have a lower risk of heart attack, in part because the omega-3 fatty acids in fish lower levels of inflammatory chemicals in the body. If you're not a fish lover, take a couple of tablespoons or four capsules of fish oil daily.

Burn belly fat Being overweight is among the leading risk factors for heart disease, and the risk is even higher when you carry the fat around your abdomen. If you have a potbelly, do everything you can to get back in shape. Losing as little as 4.5kg (10lb) can significantly lower blood pressure and protect your heart.

Don't overdo iron The risk of heart disease in women aged over sixty is drastically increased by taking extra iron. Don't take iron supplements without checking with your doctor first.

Immunity

Building your resistance

Your immune system requires a healthy diet, as well as regular exercise and adequate sleep, to repair itself and keep up your defences. You also have to cleanse your body of toxins, both natural and synthetic, that weaken your immune defences and vastly increase your chances of getting sick.

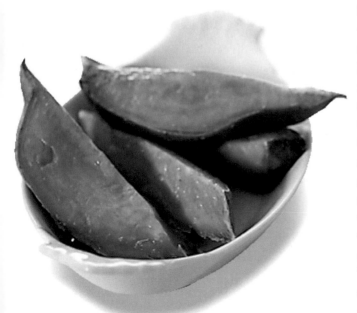

In addition to cleansing your main organs of elimination you'll want to increase your intake of core nutrients, the ones that knock out microbes and keep immunity strong.

Your detox plan

Strategy 1: Start with antioxidants

Every second, immune cells are hit by a barrage of free radicals, To stop them, take in plenty of key antioxidants.

Drink several cups of tea daily Green and black tea contain 8 to 10 times more antioxidant polyphenols than fruits or vegetables. Drinking tea can reduce cell damage caused by toxins, and help the immune system to purge free radicals from your system.

Reach for the beta-carotene The amount of beta-carotene in two large carrots is enough to stimulate your body to produce more immune cells that sweep up and destroy disease-causing microbes. Beta-carotene also dampens the carcinogenic effects of some toxins in your body. Good sources of beta-carotene also include spinach, sweet potatoes and squash.

Seek out citrus It's among the best sources of vitamin C, one of the most powerful antioxidants ever discovered. Vitamin C also may increase levels of glutathione, a compound that strengthens immunity. In addition, it helps the body to produce interferon, a protein that mops up viruses before they have a chance to make you ill.

Get E in nuts and seeds Vitamin E helps to neutralize free radicals and enhances the activity of key immune cells. Nuts, sunflower seeds and cooking oils are the best sources of vitamin E. If you're not getting the recommended 150 IU of vitamin E daily from diet alone, you'll want to take a daily supplement.

Think zinc It's an important mineral for immunity and the elimination of toxins. Zinc works with copper and manganese to block the effects of free radicals. You'll find all three minerals in most over-the-counter multivitamin supplements.

Strategy 2: Protect yourself with probiotics

Your intestine contains a thriving colony of bacteria and usually maintains a balance between beneficial and harmful species. The balance shifts, however, when your body is bombarded with toxins – from drugs, pesticides and alcohol, to name just a few. When harmful bacteria proliferate, they secrete their own toxins that can impair digestion. Your immune system gets so busy fighting intestinal bacteria that it loses strength for more important battles.

Probiotics can be extremely helpful They restore a healthy pH in the gut and boost the activity of immune cells. They also detoxify environmental chemicals along with excessive levels of hormones or metabolic by-products.

Eat more yogurt Choose those made with live cultures. Other cultured foods, such as natural sauerkraut, contain some beneficial bacteria.

Consider a supplement Even if you eat yogurt daily, you need a more concentrated source to get the full benefits from helpful bacteria. Look for a probiotic supplement that contains a mixture of species. There are many from which to choose.

Strategy 3: Detoxify your life

Detoxifying foods and herbs, along with traditional purifying practices such as saunas, are a good starting place. After that, you need to eliminate from your body and mind many of the stresses that drag immunity down.

Reduce weight People who are obese are more likely to have impaired immunity and get sick more often than those who are at healthy weights. Limiting fat intake to less than 30 percent of total calories will help to increase your immunity.

Exercise often You can't have a healthy immune system unless you do.

Give yourself some mental space If you're always stressed and in top gear, your immune system is paying the price. The important thing is to recognize when it's getting to be a problem in your life and act quickly to control it.

Menopause

Taming the transition

Conventional medical wisdom is that the discomforts of menopause are due to plunging levels of oestrogen. But oestrogen doesn't drop appreciably until after a woman's last period. During the transition phase into menopause, the time when symptoms are most apparent, women are more likely to suffer from 'ocstrogen dominance' – they have too much oestrogen relative to the hormone progesterone. This may be what causes things like decreased libido, headaches, mood swings and other symptoms.

Your detox plan

Strategy 1: Sweep out the overload

Menopause symptoms occur far less often – if at all – in parts of the world where women eat a non-Western diet and older women are respected for their wisdom. If you experience symptoms, it's essential to remove metabolic wastes or environmental toxins that could make your symptoms worse.

Drink more water You should be drinking eight full glasses a day – more if you're active or live in a hot climate.

Supplement with B complex Most women don't get enough B vitamins, a lack of which can cause fatigue and other menopausal discomforts. The B vitamins escort old oestrogen out of the body so a new supply is always circulating.

Pack in the fibre Women in their pre and post-menopausal years need to eat plenty of fruits, vegetables and other high-fibre foods. Fibre helps to pull oestrogen out of the intestine before it's reabsorbed into the body.

Take a coffee enema Coffee promotes the flow of bile and toxins to the liver for purification. For information on how to use enemas safely and effectively, see page 60.

Clear out oestrogen with soya Tofu, tempeh and other soya foods contain natural plant compounds called phytoestrogens, which block the effects of natural oestrogen and help to reduce hot flushes and other menopausal symptoms. Simply add more soya foods to your regular diet.

Strategy 2: Promote lymphatic drainage

A healthy lymphatic system is one of a woman's best friends. Here are some ways to help to invigorate your body's system.

Ease aches with castor oil In the months leading up to menopause, many women have painful uterine cramps along with headaches, fatigue and a general lack of zest – all signs that the liver isn't working efficiently. Soak cotton wool in castor oil and cover your entire abdomen, all the way around to the back. Leave it in place for about 30 minutes. It supports lymphatic drainage and helps the liver to detoxify itself.

Brush away toxins The technique, known as dry brushing, stimulates the flow of lymphatic fluid and accelerates the excretion of toxins from your body. Read more about it on pages 83 and 135.

Strategy 3: Spring clean your emotions

Clearing your body of toxins and restoring a healthier hormone balance will help your emotional balance, but you'll still need to clear out accumulated stresses and negativity. It helps to cleanse your mind as well as your body.

Take flaxseed lignans The thin hull that wraps around flaxseed is a concentrated source of a chemical compound that helps to calm turbulent emotions and also gives relief from hot flushes.

Breathe away stress Rapid, shallow breathing leads to energy-sapping build-ups of fatiguing carbon dioxide and a shortage of invigorating oxygen, along with a rise in cortisol and other stress hormones. Deep, healthy breathing exercises the organs and helps improve the elimination of toxins.

The next time you feel your stress level rising, take a deep breath, hold it in for about 5 seconds, then slowly empty your lungs. Repeat the cycle five or six times, and do it every day.

Listen to your heart A woman's menopausal years are often a time of change – changes in relationships, careers and family dynamics. Escape toxic thoughts and patterns by looking inwards and thinking about what you should be doing with your life – and how you can achieve it.

Mental alertness

Sharpen mind and memory

If you find that mental slowdowns are interfering with your ability to function normally, your body may have build-ups of free radicals, toxic oxygen molecules that damage neurons. It's also possible that your mind is filled with emotional and mental disturbances that interfere with your body's ability to cleanse itself.

Your detox plan

Strategy 1: Clean out chemical waste

Even if you eat a healthy diet, years of toxic overload can cause your body to use only about half the nutrients you take in, which in turn can leave you tired and fuzzy-headed. You can turn things around with a mind-clearing detox plan.

Cover your bases There are literally dozens of conditions, including nutritional or hormonal deficiencies, that can cause mental slowing. Thyroid disease is one, and as it is potentially serious, consult your doctor to determine whether you have the problem and how to treat it if you do.

Eliminate free radicals Your body naturally produces some free radicals, but exposure to environmental toxins vastly increases their numbers. A good way to block their effects is to get extra antioxidants in foods and supplements.

Combine vitamins C and E They're among the most powerful antioxidants, and they work best when used in combination.

Eat blueberries daily Blueberries have more anti-oxidant activity than any other fresh fruits and vegetables. The pigment that makes blueberries blue, anthocyanin, blocks an enormous number of free radicals.

Take alpha lipoic acid The body manufactures small amounts of this powerful antioxidant, but it's mainly found in foods (such as spinach, brewer's yeast and meats) and supplements. Take 100mg to 200mg daily. Other important antioxidants include selenium (100mcg to 200mcg daily) and grape seed extract (100mg to 200mg daily).

Exercise away stress hormones People who are chronically stressed accumulate massive levels of cortisol and other stress-related chemicals. Exercise reduces levels of stress hormones almost instantly, and it also gives brain cells the oxygen they need to function at peak capacity. At the same time, exercise stimulates the release of brain proteins that repair damaged neurons.

Fortify your liver Several daily cups of dandelion tea increase bloodflow to your liver and help it to remove toxins more efficiently. Other liver-protecting supplements include milk thistle and artichoke leaf.

Drink more water Get in the habit of drinking at least eight full glasses of water daily.

Eat plenty of fibre The fibre in fresh fruits and vegetables, as well as whole grains and legumes, helps your intestines to move toxins along more quickly. At the same time, fibre lowers levels of LDL cholesterol and makes it less likely to cling to your arteries and reduce bloodflow to your brain.

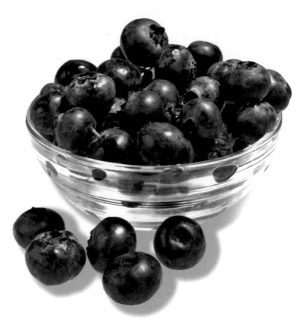

Strategy 2: Clear your mind

You can't think clearly when you're overwhelmed with negative, toxic thoughts. That's why it's just as important to purify your mind as your body when you notice slowdowns in mental energy. The breathing and meditation exercises in Chapter 7 are essential for detoxifying your mind. So are the following simple steps.

Give anxiety the boot Relaxation techniques such as yoga and tai chi have been shown to reduce anxiety and also improve bloodflow throughout the body, including to the brain.

Don't live with depression. It's the second leading cause of memory loss. And because it's often accompanied by anxiety, it can lead to elevated levels of cortisol. Try the herb St. John's wort. It's just as effective as drugs for the treatment of mild to moderate depression. Take 300mg a day. Higher doses may be prescribed by a health professional. Do not take St John's wort if you are on 'the pill', are taking warfarin or using drugs before or after organ transplantation. Hypnosis, visualization, deep breathing and meditation are also very effective ways to control depression.

Fill the air with floral scents A number of studies show that floral scents can increase learning

BANISH BRUISES

Even if you normally have good balance, there will be times when you will do something clumsy, such as smack your head against an open kitchen cupboard door. The result will be an ugly, blue-black bruise. Bruises occur when tiny blood vessels under the skin, called capillaries, leak and bleed. They usually aren't serious, but they can hurt.

To help them to heal more quickly:

Load up on blueberries They're packed with vitamin C and bioflavonoids, chemical compounds that help blood vessels to heal more quickly. As a bonus, the chemicals in blueberries make capillaries stronger and better able to resist future damage.

Pop some bromelain In addition to its ability to quell muscle pain and cramps, bromelain is like a miracle cure for bruises. In one study, researchers gave bromelain to 74 boxers four times daily. All signs of bruising disappeared in four days. In a control group of 72 boxers who got only placebos, only 10 showed similar results. Bromelain supplements are available in drugstores and health food stores. Follow the directions on the package.

speed and the retention of new material by 17 percent, probably because they promote concentration and alertness. Don't rely on chemical air-fresheners, however. A few drops of essential oil placed in a diffuser will do the trick nicely. Ask about these products at places that sell aromatherapy supplies.

Muscle pain

Soothe sore muscles

Cramps occur when a muscle contracts tightly and then refuses to let go. They rarely last more than a few seconds, but they're excruciatingly painful. Muscle soreness is a different kind of pain, known as delayed-onset muscle soreness (DOMS), it usually begins a day or two after strenuous activity.

Your detox plan

Strategy 1: Get muscles back in action

Delayed-onset muscle soreness is caused by microscopic tears in the tissues, and also by accumulations of pain-causing fluids and chemicals. You'll heal a lot faster if you pump out pain-causing substances and bring in fresh blood and nutrients.

Cold treatment At the first hint of pain, stop what you're doing, wrap some ice cubes in a face flannel or towel, and apply to the area for about 10 minutes at a time, throughout the first day. Cold causes blood vessels to constrict, which prevents pain-causing fluids and chemicals from flowing into the injured area and causing swelling.

Wrap the area Using an elastic bandage, lightly wrap the area where you have the most pain. This technique, called compression, helps to prevent additional (and painful) fluids from entering the area. However, check circulation in the fingers and toes, regularly, and loosen the bandage if it becomes necessary.

Raise it high If possible, elevate the injured area higher than your heart. This will allow pain-causing fluids to drain out, while keeping more fluids from coming in and causing swelling.

Drink a lot of water Even if you don't normally drink the recommended eight full glasses of water daily, make sure to drink a lot when your muscles are sore. Water will help to dilute chemical compounds that make soreness worse.

Take vitamin E Vitamin E helps to mop up tissue-damaging by-products that form in muscles when you've pushed them long and hard. The recommended dose is 150 IU daily.

Run hot and cold After the first 24 hours, treat the muscle to alternating hot and cold compresses. The contrast in temperatures works like a pump to increase the flow of toxins and torn muscle fragments out of the area and to bring in fresh blood and nutrients. Do this only if you have a healthy cardiovascular system. It can be risky for those with heart disease or a history of other cardiovascular problems.

Drain the fluid Once the worst of the muscle soreness is gone, gently move the injured area through its full range of motion. Moving the muscles pumps fluids and lactic acid out of the area and helps to reduce pain.

Reduce toxins with MSM While you're waiting for the soreness to fade, take a supplement called MSM (methyl sulfonyl methane), a form of sulphur that makes muscle cells more permeable and allows accumulated fluids in the injured area to flow back into circulation more readily.

Take a B-complex supplement It helps to heal injured nerve fibres that cause the pain.

Strategy 2: Take care of cramps

Since muscle cramps rarely last very long, there isn't a lot you can do to treat them. To make sure they don't come back, take 500mg each of calcium and magnesium. Muscles need these nutrients to function properly. In addition, here are a few steps you'll want to take when a cramp lays you low.

Take a grip As soon as a cramp begins, use one or both hands to massage the muscle firmly. This 'breaks up' the painful contraction and also forces out lactic acid.

Supplement with bromelain An enzyme extracted from pineapple, bromelain reduces levels of inflammatory chemicals and also flushes fluids from the injured area.

Relax in a salted bath As soon as you can, set aside half an hour to relax in a warm bath spiked with a few cups of Epsom salts (magnesium sulphate). This natural form of magnesium dissolves in water and helps to pull fluid out of the injured area and will help cramped muscles to relax.

Overweight

Purge the weight

We're surrounded by calories in one form or another, and few of us get enough exercise. But there's more to it than that. Over our lifetimes we eat, drink and inhale thousands of chemical compounds, everything from pesticides and food preservatives to secondhand smoke, many of which end up in fat stored in our bodies.

Your detox plan

Strategy 1: Eliminate toxins that trigger weight gain

One significant way to peel off the pounds and, more importantly, keep them from coming back, is to cleanse your body of the toxins that may be triggering the whole weight-gain cascade in the first place. Here's the four-step approach that may help:

1 Cleanse your colon Toxins accumulate in stools, and anything that doesn't move out of the body quickly is going to get reabsorbed into the bloodstream. For information on colonics, and more about colon health see 'Flushing the toxic colon' on page 60 and further information on pages 21 and 72.

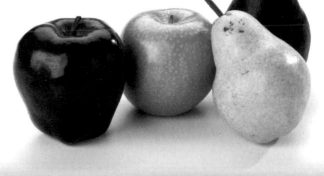

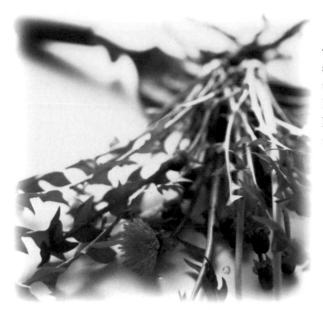

4 Cleanse your lymphatic system The lymph system pulls toxins out of cells and carries them to the liver and kidneys to be eliminated. Your lymphatic system can get sluggish when you've had an infection or eaten foods you are sensitive to. Try these suggestions.

- *Drink red clover tea* It cleans the lymphatic system and eliminates offending substances.
- *Take vitamin C* You'll need between 1,000mg and 2,000mg daily for a brief period.
- *Dry brush your skin* Use a soft brush to gently rub all over your skin, moving toward the centre of your body. Dry brushing stimulates the flow of lymph and accelerates the elimination of toxins.

Be sure to cleanse the colon and liver before detoxifying the lymphatic system. If the colon isn't moving and the liver isn't in top shape when you purge the lymphatic system, toxins will 'back up' and cause skin problems.

Strategy 2: Eat to keep weight off

Once you've detoxified your body, it's time to move to the next step of the weight-loss plan. Eat small meals more frequently. It keeps your furnace burning all day, rather than at selected times. A higher, steadier metabolism results in more calories burned.

Cut the caffeine It stimulates the adrenal glands to release 'fight or flight' hormones, which in turn shut down digestion and stimulate surges in glucose (blood sugar). This stimulates surges in insulin, which sponges sugar from the blood and stores it as fat.

Don't skip meals Even though fasting can be an effective way to purge your body of toxins, skipping meals is not. If you starve yourself, your body thinks it's facing a crisis and will begin to store fat. Studies have shown that people who skip meals tend to gain more weight than those who eat small portions throughout the day. For recipes that assist in detoxification, see Chapter 11.

2 Flush your kidneys Throughout your detox plan, drink as much water as you can. You need at least eight glasses daily. Water flushes chemicals and toxins out through your kidneys in the form of urine. Teas or supplements that contain uva ursi, juniper berry or dandelion help to flush out toxins and strengthen the kidneys and bladder.

3 Detoxify your liver and gallbladder If the liver's not functioning properly, you're going to absorb toxins that can lead to weight gain. Cleansing your gallbladder is equally important because it secretes fat-digesting enzymes. When it gets clogged with gall stones, even more saturated fat enters the bloodstream.

- *Take a liver detox formula* Many of the liver-cleansing products in health food stores contain a variety of active ingredients that help the liver to eliminate heavy metals and other toxins.
- *Take milk thistle* It has been shown to help liver cells to regenerate after exposure to cell-damaging toxins or infection from hepatitis and other diseases.
- *Think red* Beetroot helps the gallbladder to work more efficiently at digesting fats and promoting the more thorough absorption of fat-soluble vitamins.

Prostate

Detox to prevent problems

The prostate is a small gland that encircles the male urethra, the tube that carries urine out of the body. When the gland is infected or enlarged, you may experience difficulty urinating, groin pain or a burning sensation when you urinate. Preventative strategies, including taking steps to cleanse the prostate of harmful molecules or hormones that fuel tumour growth can help to ease some of the day-to-day discomfort.

Your detox plan

Strategy 1: Steps to prevent cancer

The main treatments for prostate cancer – surgery, radiation and drugs – can save lives, but they frequently cause impotence and other side effects. It makes a lot more sense for men to take the initiative and prevent cell changes that can eventually lead to cancer. Try these:

Supplement with selenium It improves the ability of your immune system to catch cancer cells at the earliest possible opportunity. It is also an antioxidant that reduces the cell-damaging effects of free radicals that are naturally present in the prostate. Taking 200mcg a day should be enough.

Load up on E It's a very powerful antioxidant that works in the fatty portions of cells. Like selenium, it increases your immune system's ability to scour your prostate of cancer cells, and it has been shown to decrease the death rate from prostate cancer. You can get some vitamin E in nuts, seeds, egg yolks and vegetable oils, but it's not enough to protect against cancer. Take a daily supplement that provides 150 IU.

Eat a lot of tomatoes They contain lycopene, a plant pigment that mops up free radicals in the prostate and appears to slow the growth of cancer cells. Ketchup, tomato sauce and tomato paste contain even more lycopene than fresh tomatoes.

Get used to tofu Tofu, along with other soya foods, contains phytoestrogens, that reduce levels of dihydrotestosterone, a steroid hormone that stimulates the development of prostate cancer. Two or three weekly servings are enough.

Cut back on fat The fat that you want to avoid is the saturated fat in milk, meat and other animal products. It stimulates your body's production of testosterone-like hormones and increases your risk of prostate cancer. It's fine to have some, as long as you reduce the overall amounts and eat more fruits and vegetables.

Go out into the sun About 10 minutes of sun each day promotes your body's production of vitamin D, that helps to block the growth of cancer cells.

Strategy 2: Slow down or reverse enlargement

If you're a man over the age of fifty, you probably have some enlargement of the prostate gland. In some cases, the gland gets so big that it presses against the urethra and makes it difficult or painful to urinate. In many cases, you can slow or even reverse this uncomfortable growth by purging the prostate of substances that stimulate the cells.

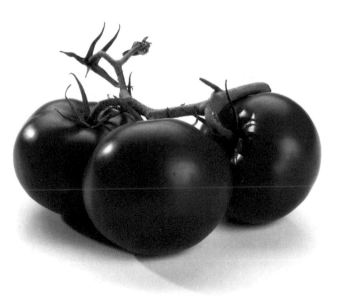

Take saw palmetto daily Extracted from a small palm shrub and available in supplement form, this herb contains a chemical compound that inhibits the action of an enzyme that converts testosterone into the 'fuel' for prostate growth.

Try nettle root It's a herbal supplement that inhibits the body's production of prostaglandins, chemicals that can flood the prostate gland and cause swelling and inflammation. If you've tried saw palmetto for a few months without success, it's fine to combine it with nettle root.

Get extra zinc It's one of the key nutrients for prostate health, and low levels have been linked to prostate enlargement. You can get plenty of zinc in shellfish, whole grains and meats. Or take a daily supplement that provides 30mg of zinc. If you do take zinc, be sure to include a daily supplement that provides 2mg of copper because zinc has been shown to interfere with copper absorption. Or look for a multivitamin supplement that contains both minerals in the correct amounts.

Strategy 3: Chase away the pain

A common source of male discomfort is prostatitis, a catch-all term for inflammation of the prostate gland. A bacterial infection can certainly cause it, but many men who have symptoms, including painful urination or groin pain, don't have an infection or any other diagnosable illness.

Prostatitis is rarely serious, but it can be extremely uncomfortable. Your best option, after checking with your doctor, is to try to flush your prostate gland of inflammatory chemicals that can cause discomfort.

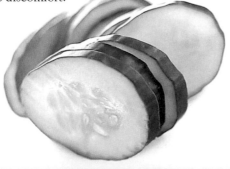

Get flower power A flower-pollen extract called Prostat has been shown to lower levels of inflammatory chemicals in the prostate gland.

Drink a lot of water It dilutes pain-causing substances and can help to eliminate bacteria and other organisms before they have a chance to multiply and cause trouble.

Try cranberry juice You can count it toward your water total, but it does more than provide extra fluids. Cranberry juice makes it harder for bacteria to cling to the walls of your bladder.

Soak away the pain Relaxing in a hot bath once a day increases circulation in the prostate, which can help to wash away pain-causing substances while bringing in healing blood and nutrients.

Eat fish at least twice a week Fish oils, which contain omega-3 fatty acids, reduce levels of prostaglandins. If you're not particularly fond of fish, take 10ml of omega-3 fish oils or two large capsules, daily.

Sexual desire

Increasing your sex drive

The introduction of anti-impotence treatments for men, and new research into treatments for women, have improved the sex lives of millions of couples. But these approaches work only for the mechanics of sex; they don't increase desire. And without desire, none of the new drugs makes a bit of difference.

Emotional issues can take the zip out of your sex drive. So can hormone imbalances or other physical problems. Scientists have only started to look at the effects of environmental toxins on sex drive but they are finding that libido is diminishing at an alarming rate. The first thing to be affected by the toxins in our lives are the reproductive organs.

Your detox plan

Strategy 1: Eat, drink and be sexy

Since medical problems are a common cause of libido loss, see your doctor. In addition, here's a cleansing strategy using food, vitamins and herbs that should restore your drive.

Follow the three-quarter rule Eat only organic foods that are free of chemical additives and preservatives, and make sure that 75 percent of the foods in your diet are plant-based foods and are eaten raw or lightly steamed. This ensures that the natural nutrients aren't removed, which gives your body the tools it needs to remove chemicals and other toxins. Natural foods are also nature's richest sources of antioxidants – they prevent artery damage that can interfere with bloodflow to the genitals.

Sip dandelion root tea A cup or two daily, combined with schisandra berries, will clear contaminants from your liver.

Clear your kidneys with cucumber Your kidneys process a tremendous amount of waste each day. To help them to work more efficiently, add half a sliced cucumber to a litre of water, and drink the water daily. Cucumber is great for detoxing because it's a very gentle diuretic.

Count on cranberry To give your kidneys an extra flush, add about 125ml (4½fl oz) of unsweetened cranberry juice to a pitcher of water, and drink several glasses daily. It helps to eliminate toxins from your kidneys, and it also promotes toxin drainage from your lymphatic system.

Knock out the caffeine Caffeine is a stimulant that can disturb normal sleep patterns without your being aware of it. Since the liver cleanses itself at night, any interruption in your sleep can cause toxic build-ups as well as fatigue.

Strategy 2: Strip away toxic thoughts

It's not a coincidence that men and women with low libido are usually stressed and tired as well.

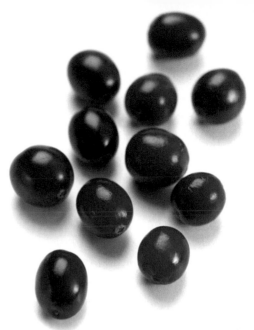

You can't have good sex when you can barely drag yourself through the day.

People breathe shallowly when they're stressed, and shallow breathing increases levels of cortisol and other stress hormones that, in turn, divert bloodflow away from the genitals. Toxic, negative thoughts are among the main causes of low libido. To get back in the mood, you first have to get out of the stress zone. Here's what to do.

Get turned on Start by turning off destructive self-criticism or mentally turning small problems into huge mental roadblocks. When you find yourself in that negative state, catch it early and distract yourself. Do something you enjoy. You'll be surprised by how easy and effective it is to turn negatives into positives.

Breathe life into your libido Even if you do nothing else, breathing deeply for a few minutes a day will strip stress hormones out of your body, improve bloodflow and help you to relax and get into the mental place where you can start wanting sex again.

Now focus on slowing down your breath. Get into a comfortable position, and breathe all the way to the bottom of your lungs. Breathe in for 2 seconds, hold it for a moment, then breathe out for 2 seconds. Keep breathing deeply in and out for 5 to 10 minutes.

After a week or two, slow the rate of your breathing even more. Breathe in for a count of 4, or even 6 or 8, and then exhale at the same rate. It gets easier with practice, and you'll find that your stress levels drop dramatically.

Skin care

Detox from the inside out

When your body is overloaded with toxins your skin does everything it can to sweat them out. As you get older, it starts to pay the price with wrinkles, age spots and loss of tone. In order to stop this downward spiral you need to purify your body as well as your skin.

The best way to regenerate tired-looking skin and take years off your looks is to start a programme that includes toxin-blocking foods along with skin-healthy herbs and products.

Your detox plan

Strategy 1: Improve metabolism and digestion

Purge with pungent spices Drinking several cups of ginger tea daily or eating pungent herbs such as basil increases metabolism and helps your liver and other organs to remove toxins more efficiently. Ginger also curbs food cravings, which means you're less likely to eat things that clog the system.
Freshen your skin with popcorn High-fibre foods like popcorn and brown rice improve digestion, which is essential for skin health because it speeds the passage of wastes through the intestine.

Strategy 2: Draw out toxins

Soothe with sesame Once a day, rub your skin with sesame oil. It pulls out toxins and makes your skin feel soft and fresh.
Soak and sweat A hot bath draws toxins in the body toward the skin's surface, and while the water cools, it pulls toxins all the way out. Adding Epsom or other salts to the bath will improve the detoxification process.
Pour water into your cells Water is almost a miracle cure. It helps the kidneys and liver to process and remove metabolic wastes. It plumps the skin and makes wrinkles less visible.

Strategy 3: Clean up the damage

Keeping your skin beautiful and clear requires periodic cleansing of dead skin cells to make room for the healthier skin below to shine through. Here are two quick ways to make yourself glow.
Use a natural peel Products that contain alpha-hydroxy acid, a natural substance found in fruits, sour milk and sugar cane, help to purge ugly, dead skin from your face.
Brush and stimulate Dry brushing may improve your skin's ability to excrete toxins. It also removes dead cells and will certainly make your skin look (and feel) fresher. See pages 83 and 135 for details.

Strategy 4: Feed your skin

Happily, some of the best foods for your skin include delicious options like fish, nuts and plenty of fresh vegetables.
Cleanse with carrots That bright orange colour comes from beta-carotene, an antioxidant that is converted to vitamin A in the body and is essential for skin health.

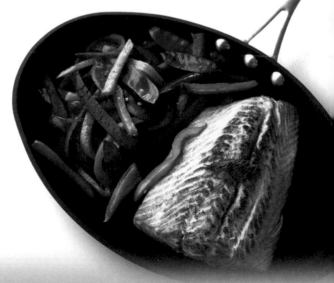

Fight wrinkles with fish Eat a few servings of fish a week. Fish contains fatty acids that reduce or eliminate skin inflammation that increases the risk of wrinkles. A diet rich in fish can also reduce unsightly flare-ups from psoriasis or other skin conditions.

Firm up with vitamin C This all-purpose nutrient is ideal for healthy, toxin-free skin. It plays a key role in the production of collagen, the protein that helps to keep skin supple and taut.

Get extra E Vitamin C is very effective at quenching skin-damaging free radicals in the watery portions of the body, but you need vitamin E to protect the denser, fatty tissues, such as those in the underlying layers of skin.

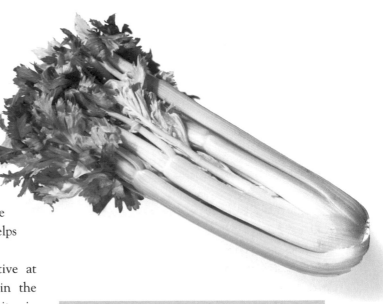

Strategy 5: Tighten your defences

There's a good reason why pharmacy and beauty stores stock so many skins creams, lotions and masks. Many of these products provide a crucial barrier against environmental toxins, including skin-damaging UV rays from the sun. If you want to ensure that your skin stays taut and glowing, here are a few things you should include in your daily plan.

Cool and tighten Skin pores act as natural traps for oil and grit. An easy way to seal out toxins is to splash your skin with cool water or witch hazel after washing.

Apply an antioxidant cream Use skin creams and lotions that contain green tea polyphenols, vitamin C or other antioxidants. They can help to prevent cellular by-products from weakening skin tissues and causing wrinkles.

Get into the sunscreen habit Too much exposure to the sun is the main cause of tired-looking skin. Your best bet is to apply a sunscreen with an SPF (sun-protection factor) of at least 15 before going outdoors.

Smoking

Curb nicotine cravings and reduce the damage

If you are struggling to give up smoking, you should at least try to detoxify your body to minimize its harmful effects.

Your detox plan

Strategy 1: Cleanse away cravings

If you've been smoking for a long time, your brain actually requires nicotine. It takes a powerful commitment to get through the withdrawal period. You can make it a little easier by reducing your body's demand for nicotine while at the same time practicing lifestyle habits that make it easier to get through those initial difficult days.

Eat organic foods Smoking lowers your body's pH, which increases the cravings. When you're trying to quit, eat a lot of organic fruits, vegetables and whole grains, and cut down on your consumption of meats and other high-fat foods. Your blood and tissues will become more alkaline, and the cravings less intense. Some of the components in fruits and vegetables bind to nicotine and help to remove it from your body.

Supplement with sulphur A product called Sulfonil, available in health food stores, binds to nicotine receptors on your body's cells. It makes the receptors less active and eventually causes cells to eliminate them. This process, called down-regulation, reduces your body's dependence on nicotine.

Optimize bowel function The longer toxins from cigarettes remain in your body, the more intense your cravings are likely to be. The most efficient way to get them out is to have regular bowel movements, and the best way to achieve that is to get plenty of fibre in your diet. You'll get enough if you make plant foods like fruits, vegetables, legumes and whole grains the backbone of your diet. You can get even more fibre by taking several tablespoons of flaxseed daily. Flax is also high in omega-3 fatty acids, which reduce the inflammation that occurs when you're detoxing.

Snack wisely Keep plenty of raw foods in the house. Carrots, celery and raw, unsalted sunflower seeds reduce the body's digestive burden and make it easier to eliminate toxins. At the same time, these snacks replace the hand-to-mouth habit of smoking and can give you a psychological boost during the most difficult days.

Create a smoke-free lifestyle Once you've made the commitment, there are ways to bolster your will power:

- *Get rid of ashtrays* and make your house a no-smoking zone.
- *Brush your teeth* often and get used to the fresh, minty feeling.
- *Stay busy* with hobbies, work, or anything else that keeps your mind and hands busy.

Strategy 2: Reduce your toxic load

The only truly effective way to reduce your risk of smoking-related diseases is to quit. But if you've only recently stopped smoking or you plan to do so at some point, it's worth taking steps to minimize the internal damage. Even if you can't bring yourself to stop smoking, you'll be healthier if you eat well and get a regular amount of exercise.

Load up on vitamin C It's a potent antioxidant that reduces free-radical damage in the lungs and other tissues.

Add vitamin E and selenium These nutrients work together to quell the harmful effects of free radicals. Selenium is especially helpful because it improves your immune system's ability to recognize and destroy the cancer cells that are caused by smoking.

Eat a lot of fresh fruits and vegetables They are loaded with chemical compounds that can help to minimize the damage caused by smoking. Those who eat fruit daily can reduce their risk of lung cancer by 55 percent.

Supplement with glutathione Available in health food stores as well as pharmacies, it's an antioxidant that improves your liver's ability to break down and remove smoking-related toxins. The recommended dose for smokers is 250mg to 500mg daily.

Take L-cysteine It's an amino acid that your body converts to glutathione – and glutathione is the most important antioxidant for the lungs as well as the liver. L-cysteine also protects your lungs from acetaldehyde, a damaging chemical compound in cigarette smoke.

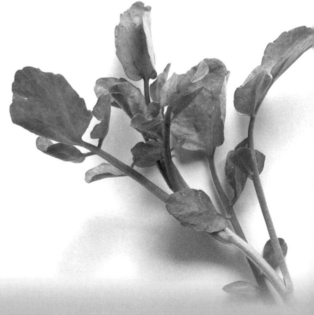

Chapter 14
Quick clean-ups
Fast and easy everyday detox tips

No matter how careful you are, you will still accumulate toxins, and they can make you sick. So it makes sense to target the particular toxin that is causing symptoms or making a chronic condition worse.

Arteriosclerosis

This is the hardening of the arteries, a condition caused by toxins, including fats, that inflame arterial walls. Here are two easy ways to keep your arteries clean and running smoothly.

Floss your teeth There is a relationship between inflamed gums and circulatory health. Some of the toxins that build up on your teeth and inflame your gums can also inflame your arteries. So take care of your teeth and gums with brushing, flossing and regular visits to your dentist.

Reach for antioxidants The antioxidant vitamins E and C neutralize free radicals. The king of the antioxidants is alphalipoic acid. Take 600mg a day in capsule form.

Bad breath

Bad breath can be a sign that your teeth and gums are in poor condition. They may also indicate that sinuses are blocked – or you may be on a diet that is just too full of strong flavours.

Open wide Pay a visit to your dentist and oral hygienist. Gum disease is not just unpleasant, but it can lead to an infection in the blood and, ultimately, heart disease. Develop a routine of brushing, flossing and rinsing your mouth after every meal. A tongue scraper will help to remove bad-smelling bacteria from your mouth.

Check your diet Try to cut down on strong-smelling foods such as onions and garlic, as well as tobacco and alcohol. Giving up milk is a good idea, too, as long as you are getting plenty of calcium from other sources.

Bladder infection

If you're fighting an active infection, you need to be under a doctor's care, but you can also help yourself by flushing out some of the toxic microbes that are causing you misery.

Juice the germs Drinking cranberry juice on a regular basis can cut the risk for urinary tract infections in half. This detoxifier works by preventing bacteria from sticking to the lining of the urinary tract, and it's been shown to reduce urine odour, burning with urination and calcium content in the urine. Do not, however, drink juice with sugar in it. Sugar can make your condition worse.

Bear with it The herb uva ursi, also known as bearberry, helps to clear the microbes that cause bladder infections. Uva ursi contains a chemical called arbutin, which has an antiseptic effect on the mucous membrane of the urinary tract. Only the leaves are used medicinally, and it's easy to make an infusion from them. Just add half a litre (1 pint) of boiling water to 25g (1oz) of leaves, let it sit for 10 to 15 minutes, then strain and drink. Or you can take it in capsule form.

Breast pain

When a woman develops breast pain, her first step should always be to see a doctor to make certain that it isn't the result of a serious medical condition. But if you suffer from tenderness and you're otherwise healthy, the problem may be due to poor handling of hormones and toxins by your liver. Here are two suggestions.

Try liver herbs Milk thistle is a great antioxidant and it helps to promote good liver function. Other effective herbs include dandelion root and artichoke, both of which increase your liver's ability to filter out toxins.

Add fibre The liver uses bile as a way to eliminate toxins from the body. When bile, which helps digest fats, is released into the intestines, it takes a toxic load along with it. When toxins get dumped into the bile, they have to travel more than 3m (10ft) to get through the digestive system. Sometimes toxins can escape the bile and get back into the bloodstream. Fibre will help to carry them out of the body more rapidly. Good sources of fibre include fruits, vegetables, legumes and whole grains. Try to eat as many as possible.

Bites and stings

Most bites and stings, which cause irritation and pain by way of toxic venom transferred to the victim, can be treated both topically and internally. However, if after a bee sting or spider bite, you notice any significant swelling, redness or have difficulty breathing, you need to seek medical treatment immediately. For minor bites and stings, here's how to clean up the venom.

Get topical Calendula and burdock creams are wonderful and calendula cream works well as a repellant. Echinacea is another excellent remedy. It speeds the removal of insect toxins from the body and quickly reduces the pain and discomfort of the bite. Put a few drops of echinacea tincture on an adhesive bandage and strapping it right on the bite. (See page 45 for more information on tinctures.)

Try homeopathic treatments Homeopathics like urtica, apis and sulphur can bring relief. Take a low-potency dose every 15 minutes for 2 hours after you're bitten or stung.

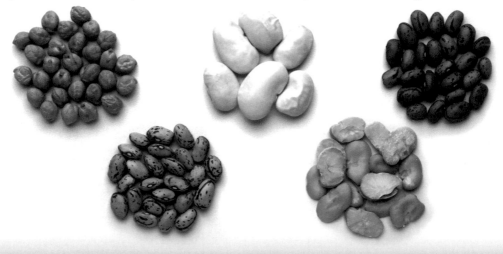

Coeliac disease

Coeliac disease is a condition that prevents your small bowel from absorbing food. The disease occurs due to damage caused by auto-immune reactions triggered by gluten, a substance in some grains such as wheat, barley and rye. If you're sensitive to it, gluten represents a serious toxic substance to your body.

Symptoms vary, but they may include pains in the gut, diarrhoea, constipation, weight loss, fatigue, anaemia and joint pain.

Detoxify your diet The way to relieve the symptoms of coeliac disease is obvious: keep gluten out of your system. Simply remove grass grains such as wheat, barley and rye from your meals. Even a teaspoon of the offending grains is enough to cause intestinal damage. Once gluten is out of your diet, your body will begin repairing damage immediately.

Play detective If you're not sure whether you have a sensitivity to gluten, you need to go on an elimination diet to determine whether you need to take the step of eliminating gluten from your diet. For more information on food sensitivities and elimination diets, see 'Sorting out problem foods' on pages 27–29.

Dandruff

The solution might not lie in a bottle of anti-dandruff shampoo.

Check your oil Body purification has two major effects: it purges the body of toxins, and it restores balance to the organ systems. If your scalp has been sloughing off a lot of skin lately, internal imbalance may be the problem, leaving your skin dry and flaky. If you have dandruff, your internal oils may be imbalanced, or you're not eating enough good ones. Try using a good fish oil or a flax seed oil, or just eat more oily fish.

Depression

Depression often indicates an overall toxic load, and studies show that aerobic exercise (walking, jogging, swimming and cycling) can be as effective as any pill. If your depression is severe, you need to be under a doctor's care. If your depression is mild to moderate, however, you may be able to deal with it on your own with these suggestions to help to lift your mood.

Lift your spirits with aminos First get rid of sugar, red meat and simple carbohydrates, which can cause mood swings. Then try a supplement of the amino acid l-tyrosine, which converts to neurotransmitters such as serotonin and dopamine. An imbalance of these chemicals in the brain is thought to be a major contributor to depression.

Get back to basics The liver is the body's most important detoxification organ, and it needs to be in good condition to deal with the general toxicity that causes low moods. So liver herbs such as milk thistle, dandelion and artichoke may be helpful. It's also a good idea to adhere to a diet rich in high-fibre foods, such as beans, fresh fruits and vegetables and whole grains.

Eat less sugar Sugar is a toxin and it's addictive. It's an obstacle to health, it stresses your pancreas and your entire endocrine system and it causes emotional ups and downs.

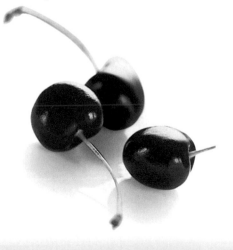

Diabetes

When your blood sugar levels are regularly too high for good health, you have diabetes. Blood glucose is normally kept at acceptable levels by a hormone called insulin, which is released by the pancreas. People with Type 1 diabetes lack the ability to produce enough insulin. People with Type 2 either don't make enough insulin, can't efficiently use the insulin they produce, or both. If you have diabetes, you need to be under a doctor's care, but there are some clean-ups you can do to help to control your condition.

Take antioxidants Take a lot of antioxidants because high glucose damages blood vessels. The damage is caused by inflammation, and where there is inflammation, there are toxic free radicals. Antioxidants include vitamins C and E. You can safely take 1,000mg of vitamin C and 150 to 200 IUs of vitamin E daily.

Manage glucose levels with gymnema Botanicals such as cinnamon, fenugreek, bitter melon and gymnema can all help to control glucose levels. But do continue to monitor your blood glucose levels to make sure they're working.

Ear infection

Otitis media, the medical term for an earache caused by an infection in the middle ear, is one of the most common conditions pediatricians see. But it needn't be. There are some easy ways to drastically reduce the amount of suffering your children go through.

Clear the air Young children who live in homes with two smokers have up to an 85 percent increased risk of developing a middle ear infection. If only one parent smokes, they have a 68 percent increased risk.

Remove milk Dairy products can make you produce more phlegm, so reducing or eliminating milk, cream and cheese consumption may help to prevent earaches. You can find a number of high-calcium substitutes for cow's milk in most supermarkets and in any natural food store. Try milk, cheese and ice cream substitutes made from soya, rice or almonds. For more information about cleansing your child's diet of problem foods, see 'Sorting out problem foods' on pages 27–29.

Flatulence

When certain types of indigestible food reach the colon, harmless intestinal bacteria break it down in a process that releases nitrogen, hydrogen and methane, as well as trace gases such as skatole, indole and some sulphur-containing compounds, which give a characteristic smell. Gas-forming bacteria feed mainly on carbohydrates and sugars. Cut down on them and you cut the amount of gas produced. The same goes for alcohol.

Fibre up Adding fibre to your diet, in the form of whole grain foods, fruits and vegetables, can help to move things along more quickly, reducing the time in which bacteria can act. Rye is a particularly good choice in that it contains more fibre than other grains do. Add fibre in small increments, allowing your digestive system to become accustomed to it.

Combine foods carefully Many people find that certain combinations of foods produce more flatulence. Eat proteins with vegetables and starches with vegetables, but never eat proteins and starches together. Don't eat acid fruits and sweet fruits together, and never eat melon with any other fruit. Drink water only after meals or about a half-hour before meals. And to make digestion easier, chew each mouthful of food at least 20 to 30 times.

Gallstones

Toxic mineral deposits in your gallbladder can be painful and difficult to treat. If your body tries to excrete them, they can get stuck in the ductwork of your body and cause a medical emergency, so prevention is your best bet.

Fatten up your food Losing weight by reducing fats in your diet may increase the risk of gallstones. To reduce the risk, add fats back into your diet in the form of quality fish (such as salmon or mackerel) and olive oil.

Gout

Gout is caused by an accumulation of toxins called purines, which form crystals in the joints, especially those of the large toe, and cause extreme pain. So try to cut the purines from your diet.

Avoid meats Purines come from concentrated sources of protein in the diet. So eliminating meats like steak, pork and lamb can help to reduce the amount of purines, which will break down into uric acid and be eliminated from the body. Anchovies, sardines, herring, mackerel and scallops also have a high purine content.

Don't drink If you have gout, you can't drink alcohol or eat white sugar, either. Beer has especially high levels of purines.

Get milk Drinking a lot of milk can protect you against developing gout. No one knows why, but presumably, milk and other dairy products detoxify the body of purines.

Get more sulphur Eat more sulphur-containing foods, like eggs, garlic and onions. Sulphur is excellent for helping the body to repair bone and connective tissue.

Heartburn

The sick, burning sensation you sometimes feel behind your breastbone is actually caused by a digestive chemical, hydrochloric acid, getting into your oesophagus. Sticking to a diet that helps your body to cleanse and purify itself on an ongoing basis (see Chapter 3) will go a long way towards helping to eliminate this problem. Here are some other ways to reduce acid.

Get aid from enzymes The sphincter muscle in your oesophagus is like a valve in that it keeps hydrochloric acid from escaping upward, out of your stomach. Sometimes it can become damaged and it allows back-flow up the oesophagus. Plant enzymes are a good a digestive aid. They work extremely well and aren't likely to cause discomfort. Bananas are thought to be a good food for this condition.

Drink lemon water Limonene is found in lemons and oranges and other essential oils. If limonene is difficult for you to find, try squeezing the juice from half of an organic lemon into a litre of water. Drop in the remains of the lemon and the peel and leave them in the water. Drink the water throughout the day in place of, or in addition to, your regular water consumption. You can even add half a cup of organic grape juice to the mixture if you find it too tart to be enjoyable on its own.

High cholesterol

Cholesterol is a waxy lipid that your body needs to make hormones, vitamin D and bile acids and to support healthy brain function.

There are two main types of cholesterol: high-density lipoprotein (HDL), which protects your arteries, and low-density lipoprotein (LDL), which can damage them and cause heart disease. Fortunately, there are some very good ways to lower LDL levels.

Eat fresh foods Drink vegetable juice, add more fruits and vegetables to your diet and drink lots of water. This will bring the body back into balance and it will begin to heal itself.

Beat it with beetroot Researchers think beetroot may work by improving the liver's ability to remove LDL from the bloodstream. It also raises HDL, and as an additional benefit, it seems to help to protect you from colon cancer.

Fight fats with fenugreek Fenugreek, a herb cultivated in both Europe and Asia, contains substances called steroid saponins, which lower the level of various harmful lipids in your blood. Fenugreek also helps to keep blood sugar levels stable in people with diabetes.

Since fenugreek is a culinary herb, you can enjoy this herb in a variety of tasty dishes. You can also take the herb as a tea or in capsules.

Impotence

If the symptom is difficulty achieving or maintaining an erection during sexual intercourse, the problem may be erectile dysfunction or, as it's more commonly known, impotence. Its causes are many and complex, not the least of which are accumulated toxins in the body. Here's how to detoxify your way to a much better love life.

Reduce free radicals Vegetables and fruits with red pulp, such as tomatoes, guavas and watermelon, all contain an antioxidant called lycopene, which can dramatically reduce free radicals that attack the prostate. An easy way for a man to get more lycopene is by simply eating a good tomato sauce twice a week.

Focus on heart health High cholesterol and smoking also greatly increase your chances of developing erectile dysfunction.

Irritable bowel

Irritable bowel syndrome (IBS) can give you symptoms such as alternating constipation and diarrhoea, flatulence, cramping, mucus-covered stool and stool mixed with undigested food. Maintaining regularity and gut health are the goals.

Bulk up Any programme to improve bowel function should begin with an internal cleansing, and one way to do that is with bulking agents. Bulking agents often contain psyllium along with other plant fibres that bulk the stool.

Eat a diet high in fibre Fibre-rich foods include beans, whole grains, fruits and vegetables. You should be doing this anyway to support your body's ongoing detoxification efforts.

For stubborn symptoms, try flax Take 1 tablespoon of whole or 'bruised' flax seed with 225ml (8fl oz) of liquid three times a day.

Bring back the bacteria Try adding yogurt containing live cultures and acidophilus to your

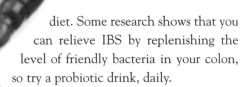

diet. Some research shows that you can relieve IBS by replenishing the level of friendly bacteria in your colon, so try a probiotic drink, daily.

Kidney stones

These stones are formed from minerals such as calcium, phosphate, oxalate or uric acid, which accumulate in the kidneys or urinary tract. Don't try to remove them with home remedies. Instead, help to keep stones from forming by preventing minerals from getting out of balance and reaching almost toxic levels.

Pile on the vegetables Just by adding more fruit and vegetables to your diet, you can halve your risk of developing stones. Switching to a vegetarian diet cuts your risk even more.

Demineralize with herbs and fruits Stones form more readily when urine stays in the system too long. A simple solution is to keep the urine flowing. An easy way to make sure that happens is to use diuretic herbal teas. Regular cups of corn silk, elder or buchu tea will do the job.

Make your body taboo to toxins Taking foods high in oxalic acid out of your diet can significantly reduce your risk of kidney stones. Foods to avoid are meat, chocolate, cocoa, sugar, sodium, spinach, baked beans, blackberries, rhubarb, peanuts, sweet potato, Swiss chard, coffee, regular beverage tea and colas. If you often use herbal remedies, avoid sorrel and yellow dock leaves, as well. Don't eliminate these foods unless you've been plagued by kidney stones in the past.

Osteoarthritis

The aches, pains and stiffness you feel in your joints are caused by joint damage and inflammation. Mopping up free radicals may help to control symptoms.

Seek out the devil Devil's claw, an herb originally found in Africa, is a powerful antioxidant that can calm down red, hot, swollen joints; reduce pain; and even bring about some improvement in the condition of your joints.

Go for E Vitamin E along with other antioxidants, lowers the risk of arthritis.

Choose cherries They contain aspirin-like compounds that reduce pain and inflammation.

Premenstrual syndrome

Symptoms occur most often at times of hormone fluctuations – puberty, childbirth, menopause or going on the pill. Fortunately, there are remedies that keep hormone levels under control.

Take the hormones out of your diet Reducing or eliminating animal products from your diet is your first step. While working on reducing your total meat and dairy intake, switch to organic farm products, which are produced from animals fed only organic feed and with no unnecessary antibiotics, hormones or animal by-products.

Chase away symptoms with chasteberry It comes in both dry extract and fluid forms. It is important to stop using chasteberry if you develop a rash. Pregnant women and nursing mothers shouldn't use it at all.

Soothe with SAMe A supplement well known for its ability to relieve depression, SAMe (methionine) can also help symptoms of PMS. Take 200mg to 400mg daily. Don't use SAMe if you are pregnant or nursing, are using prescription antidepressants, have bipolar disease or have liver disease. It is important that you take a good vitamin B supplement (containing B_6, B_{12}, and folic acid) with SAMe. Without this additional intake of vitamin B, SAMe can raise levels of homocysteine in the body, a substance that can increase the risk of heart attack or stroke.

Get up and move Exercise improves circulation, makes you breathe harder, and encourages sweating – all ways the body rids itself of waste.

Psoriasis

If you have raised areas on your skin covered with silvery, dry scales, you may have psoriasis. Normal skin usually replaces itself in about twenty eight days, but psoriasis speeds up the cycle to three or four days. Various enzymes in the liver and skin contribute to the process. Detoxifying your body and neutralizing those excess enzymes can help you keep your psoriasis under control.

Try milk thistle A psoriasis attack produces toxins, which the liver then neutralizes, so keeping the liver in peak form is essential to minimizing the effects or even preventing attacks.

Sinus conditions

Your sinuses are bony cavities around and behind your nose. They're lined with membranes that create sticky mucus when you have a cold, allergy or infection. The mucus traps bacteria and incapacitates them. When you manufacture too much mucus, however, your sinuses become blocked and can cause you miserable pain. So for relief, you'll need to clear out your sinuses.

Steam clean the toxins out A steam inhalant is a quick and effective method for draining your sinuses of excess mucus. Just add 50g (2oz) of dried thyme or eucalyptus leaves to a litre of boiling water. Remove the pot from the stove top and place it on a nonslip surface. Cover your head with a large towel, lean over the pot, and inhale. Be careful not to get your face too close to the steaming water, because there is a danger of scalding. Instead of using the leaves, you can substitute 10 drops of eucalyptus or thyme oil.

Get the mucus flowing Certain plant foods help to get mucus flowing out of blocked sinus passages. Vegetables that relieve the pressure and prevent infections from building up include onions, garlic, leeks and spring onions. Hot, fiery foods also have the same effect. Use lots of hot pepper and ginger in your cooking when your sinuses are acting up. This will relieve blockages and work to prevent headaches and infections.

Use a neti pot This is a nasal wash pot that helps to keep your nasal passages and sinuses clear of pollutants and excess mucus. For directions on how to use a neti pot, see 'How to use a neti pot' on page 62.

Stroke

Stroke is the result of an interruption of the brain's blood supply by a clot or a bleed. A diet that supports the detoxifying efforts of your body (see Chapter 3) will help to prevent strokes.

Increase fibre Eating more fats, decreasing saturated fats and avoiding salt can help to prevent a stroke.

Take some herbs Ginkgo, ginger and cayenne can also be useful. They help to stop clot formation by keeping the blood cells too slippery to stick together. They're also anti-inflammatory.

Sugar cravings

Popular weight-loss plans have prompted millions to ride the low-carb train. There's no question that these diets work, at least in the short run, but it takes will power to overcome sugar cravings. The answer is just to eat more complex carbohydrates. When you eat simple carbohydrates such as sugar, the initial energy surge is followed by a crash. Your body then craves more sugar to get stimulated again. Complex carbohydrates have a lot of fibre, so there's a slow, steady introduction of sugar into your system. The pancreas is satisfied, the liver is satisfied, and your mind is happy, so you don't crave the sugar.

Ulcers

Ulcers in the stomach and the upper part of the small intestine, called the duodenum, can be extremely dangerous. So if you have one, you should be under a doctor's care. You can, however, supplement medical care with some extremely effective detoxification techniques. The culprit behind your ulcer may be a bacterium called *Helicobacter pylori*, which embeds itself in the lining of your stomach or duodenum, causing great discomfort and and making you vulnerable to your own digestive acids and enzymes.

Help yourself by eating more broccoli. It contains a chemical called glucoraphanin, which the body turns into sulphoraphane, a very effective **H. pylori** killer. The younger the plant, the more potent it is. Broccoli sprouts contain 20 times more glucoraphanin than mature broccoli.

Urinary tract infections

Urinary tract infections (UTIs) can be painful and persistent, and if left untreated, they can lead to more serious problems. The urinary tract should be sterile; here are some ways to clean it out.

Flush your system The first thing to do is to increase the amount of water you're drinking to at least 2 litres (3½ pints) a day. The more you urinate, the less time you'll give germs to hang around and cause trouble. Cranberry juice is useful for flushing out your system, too.

Go for the green Add parsley to your diet to prevent problems from developing. Celery also helps. Dandelion leaf tea is also a good diuretic.

Yeast infections

A yeast infection in a woman is often a sign that the acid balance in the vagina has been disturbed. Here are some quick cleanups that can help you to get rid of this irritating problem.

Shift your pH If you have an overgrowth of yeast, especially vaginally, it's important to increase your alkalinizing potential. A rapid way to alkalinize is to take 50ml (2fl oz) of wheat grass juice every day, which you can find in health food shops.

Get acidophilus on your side Acidophilus can help. You can take acidophilus in capsule form or eat live yogurt.

Juice it away A general detoxification with fasting may help. For more information on fasting safely, see Chapter 6.

End the cycle Rather than treating the condition every time you get its painful symptoms, you can get at the root of the problem. Prevent these bacterial infections by raising your immune system with herbal remedies such as echinacea, maitake and calendula.

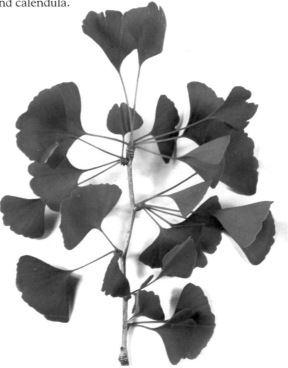

Chapter 15

Staying clean
34 steps to toxin-free living

The old adage, 'An ounce of prevention is worth a pound of cure' is absolutely true, especially when it comes to protecting yourself from the vast sea of toxins in which we swim every day of our lives.

Here are 34 ways in which you can reduce your body's toxic load in the future. Just keep in mind that the more steps you're able to implement, the less toxic your future will be and the better your health and well-being.

1 Smoke out

Stop smoking, then start eating loads of cruciferous vegetables such as broccoli, cabbage, cauliflower, Brussels sprouts and watercress. Research has shown that plant chemicals in these vegetables help to counteract cancer.

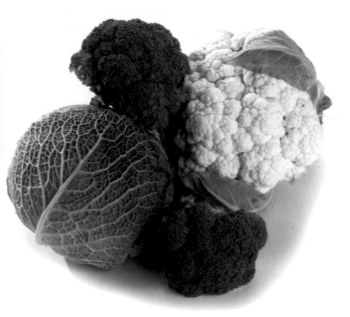

2 If you drink, do it in moderation

Indulge if you must, but when you do drink, make sure you drink at least one glass of pure water for every drink containing alcohol.

3 Control household pests naturally

Every time you spray your kitchen for ants or flies or you give the dog a flea dip, you're exposing yourself and your family to a chemical soup of poisons. Prevent pests from taking up residence in the first place. For mice, eliminate their entry points; for ants and cockroaches, keep all surfaces free of food crumbs, keep the lid to your rubbish bin tightly closed at all times and remove your pet's dish from the floor at night.

4 Use integrated pest management

Stop using garden pesticides and practice integrated pest management – it means that you don't eliminate pests entirely, you just keep them at a tolerable level and aim for a healthy garden rather than a perfect one. Many manufactured chemicals can be replaced by microbial and botanical insecticides, such as one known as

Bt (*Bacillus thuringiensis*), which are derived from plants and break down more easily in fresh air, sunlight and moisture.

5 Toss the toxic cleaning products

Take a careful look at all the cleaning products in your house with the goal of eliminating the ones that are potentially harmful.

If using slightly toxic products is unavoidable, follow usage and storage instructions to the letter, and dispose of empty containers responsibly.

Use gloves and masks where indicated, and try not to use toxic products in enclosed spaces.

6 Switch to pure cleaning power

The four best basic ingredients for less toxic cleaning are:

Baking powder It neutralizes many acid-based odours. It is also mildly abrasive.

Vinegar Vinegar kills bacteria, mould and germs.

Washing soda This is the mineral sodium carbonate. It is an excellent heavy-duty cleaner that will remove grease and even peel wax off a floor. It releases no harmful fumes, but it is caustic and you need to wear gloves when using it. If you can't find it where you live, substitute borax.

Soap or detergent Soaps and detergents cut grease and remove stains. Soap is alkaline, and detergent is usually close to a neutral pH of 7. If you have hard water, choose a detergent, as it has been designed to not react with hard-water minerals and won't cause soap scum.

7 Detoxify cosmetics

Scrutinize the ingredients labels of the products in your medicine cabinet and discard those that contain potentially toxic chemicals.

Parabens (methyl-, propyl- and butyl-) are preservatives, and they prevent the breakdown or spoilage of body-care products and cosmetics. Some people can develop skin rashes if they use or even come into brief contact with them.

Dibutylphthalate (DBP), dimethylphthalate (DMP) and diethylphthalate (DEP) are chemicals known as phthalates. These are environmental oestrogens and are linked in to birth defects in animal studies.

Diethanolamine (DEA) and DEA-related ingredients, including cocamide DEA or MEA, lauramide DEA and myristamide DEA. In 1998, a study linked the topical application of DEA and certain DEA-related ingredients to cancer in tests.

The best way to steer clear of body-care products and cosmetics that contain potentially toxic or allergenic ingredients is to watch for reactions to any new products that you try. If you experience itching, rash or skin irritations, discontinue use. If you know you're allergic to many substances, test any new product on a small patch of skin on your arm before using it.

8 Limit exposure to perflourochemicals

Minimize your exposure to chemicals known as perflourochemicals (PFCs) and in particular perfluorooctanoic acids (PFOAs), which are proving to be very persistent in the environment. They are used in everyday products such as non-stick pans, clothes that have stain protection, and personal care products. Try to use pans without a non-stick coating, and when it comes to personal care products, choose those made with natural ingredients as often as possible.

9 Pay special attention to lead removal

Although lead paint is now very rare, it may still be present in some older houses. Do not try to remove lead paint yourself. You could be exposed to dangerously high lead levels. Here are some other actions you can take:

- Water usually does not contain lead unless the home has lead in its piping. If you're not sure whether this is a problem in your house, consult a plumber. If you find lead, it's worth the expense to either have the lead removed or to buy a filtering system that will remove the lead.
- Dust and vacuum frequently as an added precaution, since lead paint is powdery as it degrades and because lead is carried into homes on shoes. Lead and other heavy metals like cadmium and aluminium are by-products of vehicle operation and are found in high levels in 'street dust'.

- Use a solution of powdered automatic dishwasher detergent in warm water to mop floors and wipe window ledges. Dishwasher detergent has a high phosphate content, and most all-purpose cleaners without phosphates won't remove lead.

10 Limit exposure to volatile organic chemicals

Volatile organic chemicals (VOCs) are gases that are emitted from liquids and solids. Common examples of VOCs include paint and paint strippers, fuels, glues, adhesives, permanent markers and even the formaldehyde seeping from pressed-wood furniture.

Choose water-based paints, stains, sealants and markers in place of those with solvents. The stronger and more persistent the chemical smell, the more likely the product contains VOCs. Choose non-toxic cleaning products and avoid all petroleum-based furniture-care products.

Make sure that there is adequate ventilation anytime VOCs are present. Another way to reduce your VOC exposure is to remove your dry-cleaned clothes from the plastic bag, out of doors, and let the clothes air before you bring them inside. This gives time for the chemicals to be released and not introduced to your home.

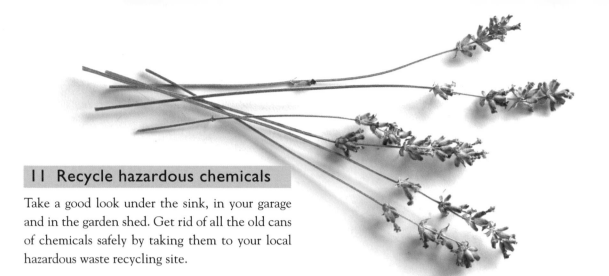

11 Recycle hazardous chemicals

Take a good look under the sink, in your garage and in the garden shed. Get rid of all the old cans of chemicals safely by taking them to your local hazardous waste recycling site.

12 Check your home for smells

What do you smell when you first enter your home? Especially if you've been away for a few days. Once you know what the dominant smell or combination of smells is, you will need to identify the source and determine its toxicity. An oil burner in need of cleaning and venting is not healthy, and if you smell strong oil burner fumes, the situation needs to be remedied immediately. The cause of mould needs to be addressed, if that is the smell dominating your home. Most importantly, use your intuition. Tend to the smells that bother you.

13 Declare war on mould & mildew

The key to mould control is moisture control. Clean any mould you find with a weak bleach solution, 10 parts water to 1 part bleach. Once you've cleaned the mould, get rid of excess water or moisture. Fix leaky plumbing and get rid of any standing water in your basement.

Three natural ingredients work very well for killing mould and mildew. The most successful is Australian tea tree oil, a broad-spectrum fungicide. Another killer, and a material that doesn't smell, is grapefruit seed extract. The third is borax, but it isn't as successful as the first two.

14 Pay attention to carbon monoxide

Don't forget to install carbon monoxide detectors along with fire detectors. If you heat your house with gas, oil or some other fuel, make sure you have a detector installed. Carbon monoxide is odourless, which makes it a stealthy killer.

15 Protect yourself from formaldehyde

Many modern kitchen cabinets are made of a plastic laminate applied over pressed wood, particleboard or plywood that could be seeping formaldehyde. The amount of formaldehyde diminishes over time, and after ten years or so the amount may be minimal. If the cabinets are older than ten years, you can simply leave them alone. You need to be more concerned about cabinets that are regularly exposed to heat.

16 Throw away disinfectant sponges

If your current sponges exude a distinctive disinfectant smell, throw them out and search for sponges made of pure cellulose. Buy only pure cellulose sponges and avoid sponges in packages that use language such as 'kills odours'.

17 Be careful with gas appliances

If you use gas, make sure that rooms are vented and that your the appliance has an automatic pilot that turns the system off if the pilot light goes out.

18 Don't heat cooking oils to smoking point

The ideal way to reduce smoke from burning cooking oils is to choose your oils carefully, cooking with oils that can handle high heat without smoking.

Also, a kitchen cooker hood or air vent is a very good way to help to reduce this form of air pollution in your home.

19 Don't eat artificial food colouring

Read product labels and avoid any product that contains artificial colours. You can make your own food dyes easily using the natural dyes from any food that will stain your clothes: blueberries, beetroot, cranberries, turmeric or even tea.

20 Get the lead out of your dishes

When purchasing new dishes, look for white china, stoneware, china without any added decorations or china labelled as lead-free. Also, avoid drinking anything stored in crystal decanters. Glass crystal contains lead, and liquid, especially acidic liquid, leaches lead from the glass and into the fluid.

To avoid lead exposure from suspect utensils and dishes, don't store food and beverages in them for longer than an hour or so. And never store acidic foods in them, as the acid will help to facilitate the lead leaching into the food.

21 Don't store or heat food in plastic

Don't use plastic containers to heat food in a microwave. Never use boil-in-a-bag foods. Avoid storing wet food in plastic. And particularly avoid storing acidic liquids, such as tea, juice and wine in plastic.

22 Protect your hands when doing dishes

Switch to a 'green' brand of washing-up liquid that doesn't have synthetic fragrances and other added chemicals. Or simply wear gloves whenever you are washing dishes.

23 Bin the air fresheners

Commercial air fresheners might smell good, but they are notoriously toxic. You can easily sweeten the smell of a bathroom by making or buying a natural potpourri or by placing a few drops of your favourite essential oil in a bowl of water to evaporate.

24 Put the lid on artificial fragrances & perfumes

Look for products that state that the source of the fragrance is an essential oil, or product labels that name the specific oil, such as 'honeysuckle oil'.

25 Don't use insecticide for head lice

The usual commercial products recommended for banishing lice may be highly toxic.

A safer (and, probably, more effective) alternative is soaking the hair with conditioner and combing it carefully with a nit comb. Add a few drops of tea tree or lavender essential oils to the rinse water. (Make sure the individual isn't allergic to the oils, and pregnant women should always consult with their doctors before using essential oils.)

26 Seal your carpets

The best wall-to-wall carpet to have is either 100 percent pure wool or 100 percent cotton. Even better, replace your wall-to-wall carpeting with hardwood floors and use cotton or wool rugs. If you can't replace carpets that are causing health problems then apply a sealant.

27 Replace polyurethane foam cushions

Ideally, cushions should be stuffed with cotton or wool batting. Polyester fill is your next best option. Have the polyurethane stuffing in your cushions replaced – it gives off toxic chemicals.

28 Cover your mattress

Replace your mattress with organic cotton, wool or natural latex, or cover the mattress with a cotton barrier cloth. Wool is naturally fire-resistant and is not chemically treated, although most sheep are regularly dipped with pesticides to control parasites, so you must specify organic wool if you want a truly pure mattress.

Encasing your mattress will help to reduce your exposure to mattress emissions and protect against small allergen particles, including dust mites and animal allergens. The cloth won't completely eliminate exposure, but it will reduce it. Don't use plastic, however. Plastic will give off chemicals. A natural cotton barrier cloth is much preferable. Do a search on the internet to find a mail-order provider for a cotton barrier cloth.

29 Scrap mothballs

Use herbal sachets to repel moths. Look for sachets made with the traditional weaver's herbs rosemary, mint, thyme and cloves. Clean all your woollens thoroughly before storing them. If you do discover moths, place the clothes in a plastic bag in the freezer for two days.

30 Don't use oil-based paints

Low-VOC (see page 180) latex paint is a much better choice, or better yet, a low-VOC paint without biocides. These are hard to find, but worth an internet search. All exterior paints have fungicides, and wood stains have even greater amounts of fungicide. The best choice for an exterior paint is a water-based paint that has zinc oxide as the fungicide.

31 Chase fleas with orange

Citrus peel extract is an excellent weapon to use against fleas on dogs, because its components kill all stages of the flea's life cycle.

D-limonene, although natural, is a VOC, so don't use it if someone in your family has asthma. It shouldn't be used around cats, either.

32 Clean up your heat source

If you heat with wood, make sure to use the most modern, efficient woodstove you can find. Avoid gas and paraffin space heaters at all costs, and make sure gas heating systems are running efficiently. Have them serviced regularly.

If you have an oil burner, make certain that it is well ventilated. And for any of these heating sources, consider having high-performance air filters installed in your home. These include electrostatic air cleaners, pleated media filters and electronic air cleaners.

A study concluded that breathing wood smoke particles outdoors on days of high pollution is equivalent to smoking 4 to 16 cigarettes a day. Imagine how much worse the problem can be indoors if your fireplace or woodstove is not properly vented.

33 Protect your family from arsenic-treated timber

Do you have treated timber in your garden, or on your deck? For that matter, has treated timber been used in your local playground? Then you should be aware that wood that has been pressure-treated with chromated copper arsenate (CCA) results in wood impregnated with 22 percent pure arsenic. This may, in the long term, be responsible for promoting cancer.

34 Repel insects with essential oils

Here's a recipe for repelling a wide variety of insect pests without chemical pesticides. (Pregnant women should consult their doctors before trying essential oil repellents.)

Insect repellent base
10 to 25 drops essential oil (see recommended essential oils, below)
2 tablespoons vegetable oil or olive oil
1 tablespoon aloe vera gel (optional)

Combine the essential oil, vegetable or olive oil and the aloe vera gel (if using) in a glass jar. Shake to blend. Dab a few drops on your skin or clothing. This easy-to-make repellent has a shelf life of around six months. If you make multiple varieties, label the jars for quick identification.

Mosquitoes Try citronella, thyme or lavender oils, alone or in any combination. (Since mosquitoes breed in stagnant water, make sure you empty all containers, such as garden pots.)

Blackflies Try lavender, eucalyptus, pennyroyal, cedar, citronella or peppermint oils, alone or in any combination.

Ticks Rose geranium is the essential oil of choice. (To protect your dog, put just one drop of oil on his or her collar; avoid using it on cats.)

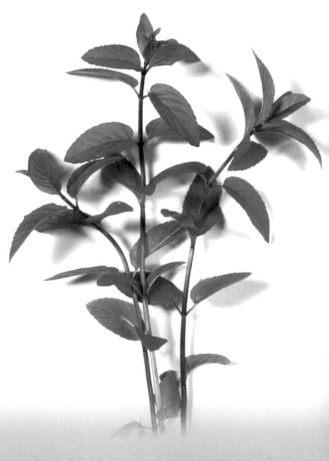

Using the recipes

The recipes in Chapter 11 assume that you are using a conventional oven. If you have a fan oven, you should follow the manufacturer's guidelines. It is usually recommended that you reduce the oven cooking temperature by 20°C (68°F) and shorten cooking times by about 10 minutes in every hour.

General observations

- Where measurements are given in spoons, it is recommended that you use proper measuring spoons.
- If you are not sure of the capacity of a cooking dish, fill it with water and then pour the water into a measuring jug. From this you will be able to judge whether the dish is large enough. If it is too small, use two dishes of of about the same size and reduce the cooking time slightly.
- Unless stated otherwise, all recipes use medium-sized eggs.
- Similarly, medium-sized vegetables and fruit have been used, unless stated otherwise.

Nutritional information

- Nutritional analyses should be used as a rough guideline only, because the nutritional value of certain ingredients may vary.
- Where a recipe suggests 'salt to taste' or 'season to taste', the amount of sodium is not usually included in the figure for sodium. But if a recipe states a specific measurement of salt, it will be included in the nutritional analysis. (To work out how much salt you are getting in grams, multiply the amount for sodium by 2.5, then divide by 1000.)
- When a recipe gives a choice of two ingredients, the ingredient listed first has been used in the nutritional analysis.

METRIC MEASUREMENTS

Because so many of the foods we buy in the UK are now sold in metric units, we have used metric measurements in the recipes. If you prefer to use imperial measurements, the conversion table below will prove helpful. Remember, though, to use either metric or imperial, and not to mix the two.

Weight		Volume	
Metric	Approx imperial	Metric	Approx imperial
15g	½ oz	5ml	1 tsp
20g	¾ oz	15ml	1 tbsp
25g	1oz	30ml	1fl oz
35g	1¼ oz	50ml	2fl oz
40g	1½ oz	75ml	2½ fl oz
50g	1¾ oz	85ml	3fl oz
55g	2oz	90ml	3¼ fl oz
60g	2¼ oz	100ml	3½ fl oz
70g	2½ oz	1 litre	1¾ pints
75g	2¾ oz		
85g	3oz		
90g	3¼ oz		
100g	3½ oz		
225g	8 oz		
450g	1lb		
1kg	2lb 4oz		

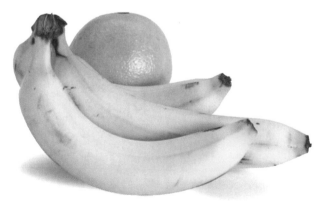

Index

immune system stimulants 39
and obesity 48
prostate cancer 163
resistance herbs 42, 43
canned foods 80–1
cannellini beans 80
chicken cassoulet 110
minestrone soup 116
capsaicin 142, 149
carbohydrates 151, 171, 172, 176–7
carbon monoxide 181
carcinogens 12, 147
carotenoids 140
carpets 183
carrots 29, 80, 156, 167
carrot-apple snazz 128
Moroccan carrot salad 124
cassoulet, chicken 110
castor oil 158
catechin 27
cayenne 149
celery 80
cells 139–40, 146
chamomile 83, 85, 89
chasteberry 175
cheese 80
barley salad with smoked cheese 120
chelation therapy 71
chemicals 44, 46, 181
cherries 175
chest press 99
chicken: chicken cassoulet 110
chicken tamale pie 111
children: ear infections 172
environmental toxins 14
child's pose, yoga 96
chlorophyll 150
cholesterol 24, 152, 155, 159, 174
cinnamon 81
circle breathing 88–9
circulatory system 19, 40, 50
citrus fruits 26, 147, 156
clay body wrap 92
clay masks 132–4
cleaning products 179
cleansers, facial 86
cleansing: blood cleansing 145–6
breathing techniques 64
colon 21–2, 60, 72, 146, 161
dental hygiene 61, 169
herbal cleansing kits 59

kidneys 146, 162, 165
Kneipp method 72–3
liver 25, 26–7, 144, 145, 162
lungs 145
lymphatic system 73, 74, 158, 162
nose 61–2, 176
panchakarma 74–5
7-day detox plan 79
skin 137, 145
see also fasting
clothes, and sweating 50
coeliac disease 171
coffee 143, 158
cognitive relaxation therapy 65
colds 40, 63, 148–9
coleslaw, Mediterranean 123
colon 10
bacteria in 31, 157
cleansing 21–2, 60, 72, 146, 161
colonic irrigation 50, 60, 72
enemas 21, 22, 50, 60, 158
exercise and 50
fibre and 139, 153
congestion, nasal 141, 148–9, 176
constipation 38, 146
cooking oils 182
copper 156–7, 164
coriander 80
Corpse pose 85
cortisol 19, 51, 151, 158, 159, 165
cosmetics 15, 137, 179
cottage cheese, berry morning crush 103
coughs 40
courgettes 80
cramps 160, 161
cranberry juice 164, 165, 169, 177
cravings 143–4, 166, 167–8, 176–7
crucifers 147
cucumber 134, 165
cumin 81
curcumin 27
curl and press 99
curries 27, 81
cushions 183

dairy products 141, 151, 172, 173
dandelion tea 38, 82, 83, 165, 170, 171, 177
blood cleansing 145

cancer prevention 147
cleansing kidneys 146, 162
for hangovers 144
for headaches 153
for mental alertness 159
dandruff 171
dental hygiene 61, 169
depression 11, 63, 143–4, 159, 171
detergents 179
devil's claw 175
diabetes 172
diaries 90
diets 28–9, 139
see also food
digestion 24, 38, 149–50
dill 81
Do-in 75
downward facing dog, yoga 95
dressings 126–7
drinks: anti-toxin beverages 47
juices 128–30
see also alcohol; water
drugs 42, 43, 46
dry skin brushing 83, 135, 145, 154, 158, 162, 166
dumbbell squats 97

E

ear infections 172
echinacea 39, 170
edamame, salted 126
eggs 80
very vegetable omelette 113
elder 40
elimination diet 28–9
emerald sesame greens 118
emotions 11, 20, 63–70
exercise and 51
menopause 158
see also mind games
enemas 21, 22, 50, 60, 158
energy boosters 150–1
enzymes 25, 26, 57, 173
Epsom salts 82, 134, 145, 154, 161, 166
essential oils 21, 133
exercise 18–19, 48–53
and asthma 140
and body fat 49
body-toning routine 93–101
cleansing lungs 145
exercise-immunology 50

premenstrual syndrome 175
stress hormones 19, 51, 158, 159,
    162, 165
housekeeping herbs 18, 35, 36–40
humming 67
hydrogenated oils 23
hydrotherapy 22, 72–3, 150
hyperventilation 67

I

immune system 156–7
    arthritis 141–3
    cancer prevention 147–8
    exercise and 19, 50
    herbal stimulants 37, 39
    immunotoxic chemicals 12
    leaky gut 27–9, 141
    lymphatic system 48–9
    natural killer cells 43
    viruses 148
impotence 174
Indian-spiced potatoes and spinach
    119
infectious diseases 39
infertility 151–3
inflammation 141–2, 154, 155–6,
    172
insects 170, 184
insulin 139, 143, 151, 162,
    172
interferon 148, 156
intestines see colon; small intestine
iron 156
irritable bowel syndrome (IBS)
    174–5
isoflavones 146

J

joints 141–3, 173, 175
juicers 29–30
juices 19–20, 29–30, 31, 56–7,
    128–30
junk food 14

K

kale, emerald sesame greens
    118
kelp powder, face mask 86
kichari 56, 107
kidney beans 80–1

chicken tamale pie 111
    Mexican red rice and beans 106
kidneys: cleansing 146, 162, 165
    functions 10
    herbal stimulants 37
    kidney stones 37, 175
Kneipp method 72–3

L

L-cysteine 140, 168
L-tyrosine 171
laughter 64
lavender oil 72, 82, 86, 87, 154
laxatives 21, 22, 33, 38
lead pollution 13, 33, 180, 182
leaky gut 27–9, 141
legs, stress relief at work 66
lemon balm 83, 89
lemons 80, 173
libido 164–6
lice, head 183
life changes, stress 66
life expectancy 139
limonene 26, 147, 173
listening to your body 58
liver 10
    cleansing 25, 26–7, 144, 145,
        162
    delaying ageing 138–9
    fibre and 24
    herbal stimulants 38
    resistance herbs 44–6
    stimulating 151
    transformers 26–7
lungs 10
    asthma 140–1
    cleansing 145
    exercise and 50
lycopene 141, 163, 174
lymphatic system 19, 48–9, 51, 73,
    74, 158, 162

M

macrobiotics 32
macrophages 50
magnesium 82, 143, 161
make-up 15, 137, 179
mandarin cabbage slaw 122
mandarin-kiwi fruit parfaits 105
manicure 88
marshmallow root tea 152

masks, mud and clay 132–4
massage 152
    Do-in 75
    hand massage 87
    Kneipp method 72–3
    lymphatic drainage massage 73
    scalp massage 89
    Shiatsu 75
mattresses 183
Mayan purifying bath 68–70
meat 142, 151, 171, 173
meditation 66, 91
Mediterranean coleslaw 123
memory loss 159
menopause 52, 147, 157–8
mental alertness 158–60
menus, 7-day detox plan 82, 84,
    85, 87, 89, 90, 92
meridians, acupuncture 75
metabolism 162
    exercise and 52–3
    fasting and 54–5
    relaxation response 63
methylene chloride 12
Mexican red rice and beans 106
migraine 153, 154
mildew 181
milk 80, 141, 169, 172, 173
milk thistle 44–5, 138–9, 144, 150,
    153, 159, 162, 170, 171, 176
mind games 79, 84, 85, 86–7, 88,
    89–90, 91, 92
mindfulness-based stress reduction
    (MBSR) 91
minerals, laxatives and 33
minestrone soup 116
mint 80
mirroring 67–8
moisturizers 86, 137
molybdenum 27
Moroccan carrot salad 124
mosquitoes 184
mothballs 183
mould 181
mouth, dental hygiene 61, 169
moving house 66, 68
MSM (methyl sulfonyl methane)
    161
mucus, sinus problems 141, 176
mud masks 132–4
muesli, fruited yogurt 104
multivitamins 26, 79
muscles: loss of 52

in food 14
in the home 15
water pollution 13, 33
trampolines 51, 93
tranquillity 88, 89
trans fatty acids 14
transformers 26–7
triangle pose, yoga 95
tuna 81
tuna tater 115
turkey, tortilla soup with lime 117
Turkish white-bean dip 125
turmeric 27, 81, 142

U

ulcers 177
urinary infections 37, 39, 169–70,
177
urination, infrequent 37
uva ursi 83, 162, 170

V

vagina, yeast infections 177
vegan diet 32
vegetables 32
fibre content 24–5
healing diet 17
juices 19–20, 29–30, 31, 56–7,
128–30
minestrone soup 116
very vegetable omelette 113
vegetarian diet 32
vinegar 81, 179
viruses, colds 148
visualizations, calming 87
vitamins 26, 79
vitamin B complex 26–7, 140, 149,
155, 157, 161
vitamin C 26
for allergies 141
for arthritis 142
cancer prevention 147
for colds 148–9
delaying ageing 140
for diabetes 172
for fatigue 151
for fertility problems 152
for heart disease 155
for immune system 156
for mental alertness 159
for overweight 162

skin care 167
stopping smoking 168
vitamin D 163
vitamin E 26
cancer prevention 147, 148
delaying ageing 139
for diabetes 172
for heart disease 155
for immune system 156
for mental alertness 159
for muscle pain 161
for osteoarthritis 175
for prostate problems 163
skin care 167
stopping smoking 168
volatile organic compounds
(VOCs) 12, 15, 180

W

walking 19, 51, 52, 92
walnuts 81
warrior pose, yoga 96
washing hands 68
washing soda 179
washing-up liquids 182
water: colonic irrigation 72
enemas 60
floral water 136
hydrotherapy 22, 150
Kneipp method 72–3
water, drinking 23, 25
for allergies 141
blood cleansing 145, 146
for colds 149
delaying ageing 139
and exercise 49
fasting 20, 55
for menopause 157
for mental alertness 159
for muscle pain 160
for overweight 162
pollution 13, 33
for prostate problems 164
thirst 144
urinary tract infections 177
weight lifting 52–3
weight loss see overweight
wheat grass juice 177
white-bean dip, Turkish 125
white blood cells 48–9
whole foods 23
willow bark 142

wine 141, 153
wood, preservatives 184
work: resistance herbs 42
stress relief 65–6
toxins 15
wrinkles 166

Y

yams 80
yarrow 83, 85
yeast infections 177
yoga 18, 19, 52
cleansing yoga series 95–6
detoxing emotions 69
hot yoga 50
and mental alertness 159
preventing headaches 154
Shavasana pose 85
yogurt 80, 150
bacteria 31
berry morning crush 103
fruit melba breakfast sundae 104
fruited yogurt muesli 104
mandarin-kiwi fruit parfaits 105
probiotics 157, 174–5
tahini dressing 126
yogurt hair mask 89

Z

zinc 143, 152, 156–7, 164